We all forget that ultimately doctors are the same as patients.

We are all veins, heartbeat, blood, emotions.

It can seem we're made of stronger, more resilient stuff.

In truth, we can be just as unsure or insecure as the next patient in the waiting room. We check our phone too much, we eat unhealthy things, we drink, we develop bad habits, we worry about friendships, relationships, family, money, the future and whether we're doing the right job both for us and for our patients.

It can take one traumatic experience,

a patient dying in front of you,

an error on your part,

a toxic work environment that makes someone leave a job,

or medicine altogether.

It's luck what situation you walk into.

brazen

Catch Your Breath

The Secret Life of a Sleepless Anaesthetist

ED PATRICK

brazen

First published in Great Britain in 2021 by Brazen,
an imprint of Octopus Publishing Group Ltd
Carmelite House, 50 Victoria Embankment
London EC4Y 0DZ
www.octopusbooks.co.uk

An Hachette UK Company
www.hachette.co.uk
First published in paperback in 2022

Distributed in the US by Hachette Book Group
1290 Avenue of the Americas, 4th and 5th Floors
New York, NY 10104

ISBN 978-1-91424-020-1

A CIP catalogue record is available from the British Library.
Printed and bound in the UK.
3 5 7 9 10 8 6 4 2

This FSC® label means that materials used for the product
have been responsibly sourced.

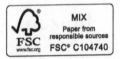

To Bobby.

To Jo.

And, of course, to Nelly.
For all the impromptu face licks.

Foreword –
A Doctor's Note

You're clearly a highly intelligent being. I mean, you're reading this book. (For which I am genuinely most grateful. Hope you enjoy it. Please tell others.) So, you'll know that prior to me writing this book in 2021 something so massive and global swamped the world with death, destruction and sheer exhaustion that barely a soul on earth hasn't been completely bombarded by it.

Or maybe you're reading this in the future as some sort of historical time capsule, wondering *how* anybody coped, or indeed can become bored of a deadly disease. Anyway, if you're feeling totally exhausted, it is mutual – I'm totally and utterly sick of Covid-19, coronavirus or whatever. Yet I've just been given a lovely engraved wooden star by the Intensive Care/Anaesthetics department as thanks for being a 'frontline hero', a nice gesture.

In the grand scheme it's like receiving a war medal on a battlefield, where the battle is still ongoing but there's an impromptu medal ceremony in the trenches. Because as I type the foreword to my book, far from this being over, we're still in the grips of a worldwide virus pandemic, currently on the rise again. A sequel in the pandemic saga is coming, and sequels are never quite as engaging as the original. No doubt they'll look at why it happened in a prequel when the franchise runs dry and let's hope it's soon.

But here's the thing, my story began differently from all this. Hopefully it will end differently too.

Some Years Ago

'Have you ever thought about medicine?' Professor Gilmore says.

'No, never. Why?'

We are chatting over the contents from a large hydatid cyst in the London School of Hygiene and Tropical Medicine (LSHTM) laboratory, taken from the abdomen of a patient who had eaten a dog tapeworm during a meal some years ago, presumably by accident. It looks like one of those sad, saggy old balloons after a birthday party, except this one is full of rancid parasitic pus. The surgeon's aim is to remove it intact. If it bursts inside you, the contents are splashed across your insides, causing massive anaphylaxis and death. It is taken out carefully by the surgeon, hopefully with minimal hand tremble. Luckily this one had kept its football-sized skin intact until outside the body.

'Oh, a fine specimen!' Professor Gilmore says excitedly. 'It'd suit you.'

'Medicine or the cyst?'

✛

I didn't take the straight path to becoming a doctor, more the scenic route with stops along the way. As a budding parasitic student (like all students), medicine had never really occurred to me as a career, but the thought of becoming a doctor began to burrow its way into my brain.

I never thought anything would usurp my love of parasites. These individual monsters of varying sizes are so much more exciting than a bacteria or virus. Parasites have personality, they feel exotic, probably because you find a lot of them in exotic climes. I study everything from toxoplasmosis (spread through cat poo), pinworm (which causes the classic itchy bum) and malaria (the same thing Cheryl Cole had) to river blindness (a worm that makes you blind), schistosomiasis (or Bilharzia, the 'gap-year' ailment) and Chagas disease (spread by insects that kiss you at night), even forensics and the bugs that colonize dead bodies. I love being in the school's old laboratory, with its wooden benches, characteristic smell and various instruments and apparatus. The microscope is the main tool here, basic but effective, especially in a developing country where resources are scant. Now, by looking down a microscope at a blood film, I can tell you not just whether a patient has malaria, but *which* type of malaria it is. Who doesn't appreciate that little party trick?

The school's John Snow Society was named, not after *Game of Thrones*, but after the physician who, in the 1800s, found that cholera cesspits leaking into London's water supply might actually, you know, be the cause of the cholera outbreak. The research I was doing for LSHTM wasn't a million miles away from that; in fact, it was only several thousand away, in China.

If looking at intestinal worms in kids doesn't sound appealing, the actual groundwork is worse – collecting faeces from schoolchildren. It sounds like the kind of project that wouldn't take off in the UK, but would probably make the news. Staring out at the clouds from the airplane, I still have no idea how the samples will be collected until I arrive in China. The officials there clear this up. They want me to speak to classes of children, in a Western-man-on-his-gap-year style, except instead of 'finding myself' or building a school, I am to ask every child to please go home, defecate in a pot and bring it to school like some sort of show and smell. At the first school we visit, a teacher and I stand at the front of the class, and due to my lack of lingual skills I explain in English:

'Hi, everyone, I'm Ed. So I'm doing some experiments looking at poo and I would love it if you could all take one of these tiny cardboard boxes . . . '

Why are they cardboard? I think.

' . . . and, well, poo into them, then bring them back to school with you. Unless you poo here of course . . . '

Silence and stares. The teacher looks at me sternly, then says something to the official who drove me out here. I can't understand the language, but I'm pretty sure it was 'Is this guy for real? Is this a joke? Do the authorities know this crazy English man is going around collecting children's POO?'

The teacher side-eyes me while translating my request.

But we have LOTS of donations over the next few visits, children enthusiastically bringing pots of poo to me, sometimes with the lid not firmly on. For the next eight weeks in the local laboratory, I live the life of a crap-collecting hermit, with a microscope and a faeces-filled fridge, which is nonchalantly used by other staff to store their lunch.

Before I leave for China, Professor Gilmore, who was not content with my shit workload, says he wants me to bring back souvenir samples for the lab in London and proudly presents a letter of permission from the university and some 'airtight' containers.

'Just wrap them in some clothes, they shouldn't leak.'

'Shouldn't' wasn't reassuring. One thing worse than bringing faeces back in my backpack is faeces *leaking* in my backpack. I pray for a gentle-handed baggage handler, and apply to study medicine on my return.

China is on my mind for another reason too. Our last class assignment was a hypothetical disease-outbreak scenario, starting in rural China and subsequently arriving in the UK. We had to gather symptoms and trace contacts, conduct surveys with actors, calculate infection rates, make recommendations and file a report within 48 hours. We needed to work fast. Over the scenario, new outbreaks occurred and curveballs were thrown in by tutors. It was dizzying, caffeine-fuelled and ultimately a success. My contribution of Jaffa Cakes to the group was no doubt an absolute game changer to our energy, undoubtedly saving countless theoretical lives.

So there is an oddly familiar sense that years after my outbreak scenario at LSHTM, I'm now a doctor, an anaesthetist (anesthesiologist), on the so-called front line, facing a pandemic outbreak where hygiene is important. People in the upper echelons of government no doubt have a crisis task-force group, like us on our assignment. I remember that strong leadership, acting early, clear communication and planning were key to overcoming it. If a bunch of course students can manage it, surely a real government with money, experts and resources would? We are safe in Boris Johnson and the UK government's hands, right? Maybe someone forgot the Jaffa Cakes.

✛

You may have already made the connection between anaesthetics and coronavirus, but if not: coma-inducing drugs, patients not breathing for themselves and ventilators are all to be found in Intensive Care Units (ICUs), where the effects of Covid-19 have hit hardest. Back in the day, in the UK at least, an ICU was staffed almost exclusively by anaesthetists, before it became a separate specialty in its own right. Nowadays all anaesthetists do still train there and indeed staff them overnight or on call, because there just aren't enough doctors trained to look after people's airways. Many anaesthetists leave it behind after their duties through training come to an end. There are several reasons why: it can be exhausting, sad and incredibly draining, plus it's very different from anaesthetics day-to-day. Anaesthetists tend to take patients off ventilators so that they can go home. In an ICU, it can be to live or let die.

So when Covid-19 struck, a disease that affects your breathing so badly that you need ventilating, and with limited ICU capacity due to the chronic underfunding of our health service, there was an army of nervous anaesthetic trainees, like me, drafted into ICU front lines. Whereas our A&E (ER) department enjoyed less footfall in the first ever lockdown, just a few steps away my anaesthetic colleagues and I were sweating away in a makeshift ICU, where enabling people to survive a few hours was a success. In my hospital, it was mainly the trainee anaesthetists or staff grades. Anaesthetic consultants who were not already working in ICU were largely protected and ran whatever surgery we could keep going, leaving us younger, supposedly less at-risk ones to the front line. Yet there are only so many of us, so doctors from other specialties were drafted in to help and anaesthetists were rationed across the rota to ensure there were always some airway doctors on.

I don't know if I'm allowed to say this in a book, probably not at the beginning, but I'll be honest with you. Despite being in the thick of this pandemic in the NHS, there's a part of me that feels completely inadequate, unqualified even, to tell a story that I was wholly part of. A first-hand-witnessed account, yet am I fit to tell the story? I don't know if it's pathological of the whole scenario, where feeling helpless became the new norm. Facing a deadly disease that you and even your seniors are oblivious to, hearing news reports from abroad telling you more than medical training, the horror of every day not really knowing what you're doing or treating. We create guidelines and strategies to follow, to keep safe. But they're just guidelines, not rules, and no one knows the rules of Covid-19. Maybe those processes and guidelines are simply to stop us going mad. ICU became a minefield where anything you touched could lead to death, a constant gripping anxiety. Thirteen-hour days, with a one-hour commute, left me nine hours to eat (one hour), stare at the TV/phone/wall (two hours) and sleep (zero to six hours, depending on anxiety levels). I told myself I was OK, getting through it. But the candle quickly burned through both ends and only now do I realize that. During full lockdown, I assumed the freedom of working in hospital would make life easier. But it was more prison to day-release prison and back.

Of course, pre-pandemic I had difficult days/nights in hospital too. But my usual coping mechanisms, like many other people's, disappeared overnight. My mind fluctuated, I thought that I'd lost it on a number of occasions. I became acutely aware of the hospital, the building and its structural failings, what with all the time spent staring at the walls. Every hospital I've worked in seems to be crumbling. As you go through the gears from medical school to junior doctor to consultant, you naively believe things will improve, structurally and practically. But over time, you realize that things won't change. Why are we still using crappy IT systems that take ten minutes to log in? Why are NHS staff paying for parking? Why isn't there sufficient local-transport infrastructure for health-care workers? Why can't they provide food for workers forced to use food banks or pay them more? The reason why NHS workers are 'heroes' is simply due to the conditions we find ourselves working in, not our jobs.

I digress. Let me tell you how I ended up here.

Chapter 1

Anyone can be a doctor. OK, not *everyone* but, you know, most people *could* be.

One of my best friends recently called me after his wife gave birth in hospital. He was drunk on endorphins and telling me about their baby, the delivery, but most importantly their anaesthetist.

'They were incredible, just fantastic! Then I remembered, Ed, *you're* an anaesthetist . . . Fucking hell! I can't believe that . . . no disrespect . . . *you've* got that responsibility.'

I like to think I'm an inspiration to all budding doctors that anything is achievable. No matter how late you choose.

✚

I secure my place at medical school so late that I join a mass of new University of Aberdeen recruits without accommodation, so my second Freshers' week starts in a Premier Inn, which is actually comparative luxury compared to student digs. My first friends are other Premier Inn outcasts and after nights out we hang in the hotel bar like the last guests at the wedding. When I finally move into halls and restart the friend-making process, I have a fair heft of impostor syndrome, as people already know each other. Trying to get to sleep on my uncomfortable new bed, I know how much first impressions count, so I plot how to get off to a good start here.

This is when Mum calls.

'Mum, it's 11pm. Why are you awake?'

'Ted, you need to go to the supermarket.'

'What, why?'

Mum tells me urgently that there will be a run on food tomorrow due to the swine flu outbreak news.

'It's going to be in the newspapers tomorrow, we've stocked up, you should go, now!'

Never has my mum exaggerated, *never*. Always the voice of reason, and a total sense of calm. There's a famous adage in medicine to *always* be worried about the farmer with no past medical history who turns up to see a doctor, because they wouldn't normally make a fuss. This feels similar.

I pull some clothes on and leave my room. Suddenly I'm filled with guilt about my fellow soon-to-be-starving students. What if they need something? I decide to knock on each door.

'Hi. Listen, don't tell anyone . . . but I'm going to the supermarket. Do you want anything?'

All of them look bewildered before thinking I am pulling some kind of joke. I try hard to assure them that my mum is never wrong on these things, but I can't raise their levels of concern. I return just after midnight with bags of panic-bought tuna, pasta and mayonnaise. Survival will taste dull, but survive I will.

The next day, nothing, no panic. Nothing in the news either. I look outside and there is no one from the university advising people. A text arrives from Mum.

'False alarm, so sorry for calling late. Hope you're having a great time! x'

'Ohhhh, shit!' I say out loud.

I walk into our shared kitchen where everyone has already seen the huge mass of tuna sitting on the worktop.

Outside, word spreads and for my first few weeks I am known as that crazy Swine Flu Tuna guy.

✚

There's a unique mystery to starting medical school. On one hand you learn in depth about human physiology and disease processes, on the other you spend a lot of time with dead bodies.

Body donations these days are sometimes so frequent that anatomy departments have to turn them down, or even turn donations down because of the day you die. Since bodies need to be received within 48 hours of death and anatomy offices are closed at weekends, dying on a Thursday or Friday can rule you out. The same goes for Christmas and New Year. Death needs to call back between 9 and 5pm, Monday to Wednesday and when Santa isn't around.

Most people remember the first time they ever see a dead body. For me, it's on my first day in Anatomy. Classes are held, for the last *ever* year, at Marischal College in Aberdeen. This huge building is not only the second-largest granite building in the world, but was also purported to be Hitler's favourite building in the UK, apparently a rumour made up by students decades ago, *apparently*. Still, as the only students entering through the back door into an eerie, frosty, grey stone courtyard, you can more than believe it. The anatomy staff know this and attempt to accustom us to the odd learning environment by laying out an entire dead body for our arrival, along with some other dissected body parts. We all mingle about, looking and nodding thoughtfully, wondering who will be first to mention the terrifying dead body in the room. The smell of embalming formaldehyde is rank and everywhere, intensifying all the body parts and anatomy tools. I look at the body, a bald, elderly man, and notice something strange. It is complete except for the genitals. What is the reason for this? Were the genitals not donated along with the rest of him? Were they stored elsewhere?

'Could it be a dying wish?' Max, a friend that has lasted past Freshers' week, says.

'What? A dying wish to have your balls cut off?'

'Hmm, maybe not.'

We finally decide to ask the person in charge, Professor Yates, head of first year.

'Excuse me, Professor, we were just wondering why the penis and testicles have been removed from the body?' I gesture across, in case he hasn't noticed the dead body in the room.

I feel happy that we aren't squeamish, acting like sensible medical students. Dr Yates' eyebrows raise in an impressed manner of 'what a very good question!' I let a dream swim before me: this will be the start to an exceptional first year, where I'm well regarded among the teaching faculty, with possibly even a distinction at the end. When they present it to me, they will pat me on the back and, out of earshot from the other students, confide: 'We knew you were special when you made that observant remark in your first anatomy class.' I will return a knowing smile and we will file out of the lecture theatre in professional silence. When I suddenly see Dr Yates' face contorting from pride into astonishment, my golden future looks to be shifting further from reality. He looks around, then at me and Max, then at the body, then to me again. His face settles on puzzlement.

Taking a slight cough, he clears his throat.

'That's . . . a female and that's . . . a vagina.'

I suddenly become very hot. Very hot indeed. Sweat manifests itself from places I didn't even know sweat glands existed, ready and waiting in silence, all my life, to reveal themselves at this very moment.

'We . . . just shaved the head. Did . . . did you not think about that first? Before asking who had mutilated a dead person's genitals?'

I was rosy by this stage and glistening like a disco ball in the light.

Professor Yates looks around the room to see if he is being filmed for a prank, or whether security has accidentally allowed a non-medic in. Max stares at me, hoping I have a way out of this.

'Oh, yes, well . . . ' I say, trying to sound calm, ' . . . I've never seen . . . a vagina before.'

Dr Yates raises his eyebrows again.

Nothing has ever felt this awful since my parents gave me business cards for a 16th birthday present, with my picture, home address and landline number, telling me it will help me make friends at my new school. I have no friends from that school.

As a medical student it's normal to spend half a day around dead body parts. It helps you become acclimatized to the formaldehyde, which also has a side effect of making you incredibly hungry, then nauseous because of what you're looking at, then hungry again. Sort of like having food poisoning but without the release.

When not dealing with dead bodies, I am, perhaps even more uncomfortably, dealing with alive ones, mainly classmates. Clinical skills sessions require learning the systems and examinations in working bodies – the lungs, the heart, the abdomen, etc. You practise and learn on each other. Luckily, there were always people willing to be examined, mainly because it means you get to lie down for a bit. First-year medical students are *the* most experienced at examining people with hangovers.

Now, of course, there are some things you obviously wouldn't examine on classmates: rectal or genital exams are a no-go. So instead, these are talked about in theory and then we practise on models, which sadly aren't the best, because no matter how much you try to believe that a pair of rubber buttocks in front of you is a patient and address them with 'Hello, Mrs Brown, I just need to do a rectal exam . . . ', it just never feels convincing enough. For instance, I almost always forget to put on gloves to insert my finger into the Mrs Brown model, but I guarantee you that is the *first* thing I'd grab in real life – hell, I'd even double-glove.

After learning on each other and the odd Mrs Brown model, we are allowed to move into hospital to try out both our new skills and name-engraved stethoscopes on real patients. Patients are usually amenable to students, but if someone has interesting chronic signs or a heart murmur, it often results in a consultant and around ten excitedly apologetic medical students all crowding into a cubicle, desperate to get experience and exam practice.

Outside of medical school, I throw myself into undergraduate lifestyle and counter impostor syndrome, going from steady adult life to doing Jägerbombs on a Tuesday night around Belmont Street in the city centre, where students and oil-rig workers party side by side. Even my relationship goes the way of most pre-university romances, splitting up with my girlfriend shortly after starting medical school. Keen to spread my social wings, I take up Ultimate Frisbee, a very 'university' activity that attracts a mixture of characters, some of whom take it *very* seriously. It's a sport yet to gain much UK traction outside of university circles, the exception being on my nipples. One afternoon, a mixture of cold Aberdeen air, rain, a nylon top and a lack of base layers results in much chaffing. Sore and now late back from training, I don't have time to shower before a tutorial, so instead I pull on a shirt and run to hospital. I have no idea why my classmates are silently gesturing until the person sat next to me gasps and I look down. My nipples are bleeding through my shirt. Humiliating at the best of times, even more so in a tutorial on breast cancer.

✚

As I slip through the gears and years of medical school, I start thinking about what specialty I'm heading for. I have no strong feelings, but I'm pretty sure it isn't going to be surgery. I tell this to my dad, who needs an operation to repair an aortic aneurysm.

'Apparently I need a vascular surgeon. Could you do it?' he says.

'Probably, but I wouldn't rate your survival chances after, or during.'

An aneurysm is a widening of the blood vessel, in this case the biggest artery in the body, the aorta. If it bursts, the chances of surviving are much worse than planned surgery. That being said, it's still a high-stakes procedure and is only done when the risk of bursting outweighs the risk of surgery.

I head back to Nottingham and see Dad before he heads in for his operation. There is still a risk of things going wrong, so a few nervous hours are spent pacing around before he's out and into the high-dependency unit. We visit the hospital and, among the family relief, I notice that I am pretty much lost in the surrounding clinical environment. I naively assumed that having now been in a hospital, I'd find this one all familiar and comfortable, but I don't. The general set-up is the same, but I don't recognize anything – the equipment, monitors, computers – everything is slightly different. This is the moment I realize they are absolutely not the same: every hospital will force me to learn afresh.

✚

After Dad recovers, I head back to Aberdeen, although not for long. A General Practice (GP) rotation means I am sent to Castle Douglas, a small semi-rural community where everyone seems to know or be related to one another. I join the local practice and live with a couple of other students in a B&B. My room was advertised as a four-person room, yet I have it to myself. What junior suite is this, I wonder? Is there a minibar and an indoor hot tub? It turns out to be a dank double room, with four single beds crushed inside, leaving little room to move or store anything. But it does mean falling out of bed results in falling into another bed. The collective noun for doily mats is something I could do well knowing, as is a conversational level of DIY-ability, since most of the lights have no bulbs. All good experience for NHS on-call rooms. One thing you cannot fault is the hearty breakfast served each morning, a daily intake of fried breakfast at 6am. There is no menu, it's just presented to us as a fait accompli. Eventually, we gently request less and less, until a single piece of toast is provided.

One evening, we plan a night out in local Dumfries.

'Dummmfries!' booms Dr McBride, one of the General Practitioners (GPs), as I tell him of my plans.

'Hang on there, laddie.'

He goes next door and comes back with a brown paper bag.

'Well, then, you'll need these.'

Inside are 12 condoms.

'I don't think . . . '

'Yer can never be too careful,' he says, coming close to my face and wagging a finger.

If nothing else, he was painfully optimistic.

✚

My time in Castle Douglas is followed by my elective placement. This gives medical students the opportunity to go anywhere in the world and gain experience of different health-care systems, in both developing and developed countries: it's your choice to organize. I decide to look at skiing and snowboarding injuries, because I really want to save the world from middle-class injuries. After managing to sneak onto a fully booked rotation with the promise of bringing some whisky, I head to Montana, USA, where, for six weeks, I spend half a day working in the GP practice on the slopes and the other half playing in snow. It is slightly different from Castle Douglas: I have to ski to work each day and people pay for health care. It is such an odd change – seeing people pay for medical treatment, that is.

As someone brought up on health care being free at point of use, a human right, it is a completely different culture. Money matters. As the only British student there, I watch conversations about which specialties people will apply to, similar to conversations I have, but with a key difference being how much money they will make in their chosen field. In the UK, no one chooses medicine to make a lot of money; there are much better paid and perked jobs out there. GP is one of the most popular medical jobs for lifestyle in the UK, building rapport with patients and a love for primary care. In the US, at least for some, family medicine is discounted purely because it doesn't make the best money.

Medical exams are like nothing I've done before, but they represent the nature of exams we'll take for the rest of our doctor lives. Yes, exams don't stop when you become a doctor, as you shell out exam fees again and again to make it to the next levels of your career. Eventually they stop, when you retire. Observed Clinical Structured Exams (or OSCEs for short) are the practical exams. Essentially, they have around 15–20 stations, each like a mini escape room, where you enter a curtain to find a variety of challenges – a patient to talk to or examine, a test to conduct, results to interpret, a mannequin to do chest compressions on or similar. Some of the actors would put on the tears and provide Oscar-winning performances of upset or angry patients.

It's an exam in which you can never be *fully* sure how well you've done. During one OSCE, the examiner asks me to examine and listen to the patient's heart sounds. I go through my routine and haphazardly pop my stethoscope onto his chest to listen to the heart. As I place it in the different regions on his chest, each time I hear absolutely *nothing*. Is my stethoscope broken? The examiner asks me to present my findings.

'I . . . I found it difficult to hear . . . anything . . . anything.'
'Really?'
'Yes, I cannot hear this patient's heart beating.'

This raises eyebrows from the patient who was looking very alive. The examiner asks me nothing more, looks low and scribbles on the mark sheet.

I write that station off, but when the results come back, I have scored full marks in that station and much less in the ones I thought had gone well. So, either that patient has dextrocardia (the heart is on the right instead of the left side) or the mark sheets got mixed up.

✚

The other exams are written, mainly single best answer (SBAs) with a few short answer ones, although the short answers are being phased out, either due to marking being easier by machine or to prevent medical students showing off their uninformed guesswork. One exam question asked 'name a treatment for mastalgia' (breast pain) and it was estimated that around 80 per cent of male students in our year wrote 'massage'. Thus, SBAs are fast becoming the popular exam, where a question is followed by five possible answers: any could be right but only one is the *single best*.

You quickly learn that anything definitive is generally incorrect. If a question or answer contains words such as 'never' and 'always' you know they are false because real life has caveats and anomalies, there's *always* an exception. It's a technique that becomes ingrained in medical professionals taking these types of exams. If an exam question were to ask 'Is the anus *always* outside the brain?', doctors would confidently answer 'False'.

Despite my previous experience with exams, these are in a totally different league of difficulty and dread-filling, with the added pressure that every exam counts towards your final-year ranking and chances of getting a doctor job. They require a vast amount of knowledge that is direct and precise, leaving no room to reason hypothetically. If asked what is causing someone's central crushing chest pain, replying 'Maybe someone is sitting on their chest?' won't win you points, fans, or a General Medical Council number.

Eventually, I, like everyone else, become a panic-stricken hermit, surrounded by non-medical student friends lapping up the freedom I no longer have. It's impossible to keep hold of all the knowledge, it drips out of you like a leaky brain faucet and you only retain information you need or use, or random facts that have clung on to your brain fibres (see, scorpion stings cause pancreatitis). Even in hospital, when close to exams, doctors will turn to medical students when faced with unusual questions or diagnoses.

'You're doing exams soon? Well, you should know about this?'

➕

I am not top of the year, far from it. Although one blue moon sees me excel in a single exam after I assume, like *all* annoying people who do well, that I'd done extremely badly. In my defence, immediately afterwards Max pointed out the – now *obvious* – correct answer for a question that I had got completely wrong. So being the optimist, I assumed failure for the rest of the paper. To my surprise, I receive an email saying quite the opposite, instead asking if I would return to Aberdeen for a prize interview. A prize! Nothing like this has ever happened to me before.

This chance of a prize means getting a last-minute eight-hour train back to Aberdeen. On the way up, my mind yet again turns to dreams of glory, entering the history books of prizes. I have my best (and only) suit to match my haircut and shave. After being quizzed in a relaxed prize-interview format by the panel of three consultants, I meet Max for a beer, then head to the station the following morning. At 8am, hoping for a quiet return journey, I spend the eight hours home sat in a train carriage full of oil-rig

Chapter 1

workers, who have just come ashore and started drinking heavily. Two days later, a letter arrives. Excited, I open to find . . . I've won!

I read out the letter to my excited parents.

' . . . and we are delighted to announce you are *winner* of the prize, enclosed is . . . '

'What? What is it?' Mum says.

' . . . a cheque for £60.'

'That's not bad!' says Mum.

'Not bad?' I say exasperated. '*Not bad*? Sixty. Pounds? It cost me £84 for the train ticket. Meaning my prize is what? Minus £24 plus 16 hours of train journey.'

'Well, we're *very* proud of you.'

At least, I've come a long way from being unable to recognize a vagina.

✚

After passing my final exams alongside crushing anxiety, medical school leaves me on a high, followed by lasting reminders that it doesn't teach you everything and there's much still to learn. This was demonstrated in clinic with a consultant who caught me off-guard.

'Ed, would you like to examine this gentleman's testicles?'

The use of the word 'like' never failing to catch me by surprise.

Fortunately, he was gesturing to someone who appears to be a patient, not a random person. So I feign great enthusiasm.

'Yes, I'd *love* to.'

Love to?! Too much feigning, Ed, way too much.

It is a nanosecond later that my brain triggers a realization that I've never done this examination on a patient before. Sure, I'd used the Mr Thomas testicle model, but that was *just* the testicles as a hanging appendage, similar to a bunch of low-hanging fruit. These testicles are attached to a human. How best to assess them when they're not at table height?

Seconds later, with the word 'love' still swimming in the ether between us all, I proceed to do something that will stay with me for the rest of my life and just saying this, writing these words, brings back a ripple of PTSD so strong that I feel queasy. So please, dear reader, take a deep breath and understand I share this with you so that if ever you become a doctor and this situation arises, you know not to follow in my path.

I did what you should *never* do.

✚

I got on my knees.

Once the bend at my knees begins, I realize this is a terrible, terrible mistake, but I can't stop mid-squat. In the small consulting room, I panic-turn my head beseechingly to the consultant while continuing to lever myself further in the downward motion. Wait, did something just brush my cheek? Suddenly I feel sick.

I gently and reluctantly examine the testicles, trying to keep a professional face.

'I think I'm done,' I say to the consultant a few seconds later, a penis hanging right between my eyes. I feel like Liam Gallagher when he addresses the microphone. After the consultation finishes and the patient leaves, the consultant closes the door and solemnly turns to me.

'You know Ed, next time, you probably shouldn't get on your knees.'

Like I *need* to be told.

✚

My final months as a student are spent on a surgical ward. It is also where I first see a death certified by a doctor.

'Ed, do you want to join me?' offers Zak, one of the hospital's junior doctors.

I have never seen someone in hospital who's died. We enter the side room, where a calm and quiet atmosphere surrounds us, the patient motionless on the bed. Zak does some checks, then places a stethoscope, listening to the lungs while feeling for a pulse, his head hovers above the mouth listening for breath sounds, all the while watching the chest. Sadness creeps over me seeing this life has ended; this person will have had hopes and dreams like the rest of us, all of a sudden gone. The impact is not just on them, but their family, their friends and more. Like blood vessels, one life connects others by many routes that we don't always understand. Zak's checks last for several minutes before he quietly nods to the nurse, then me, and we leave the room. We're silent in the corridor, it's affected me more than I realize. Finally, I break the silence.

'So, did you hear anything?'

'No, of course not, you idiot.'

Chapter 2

I constantly think back to my ineptitude with those testicles. And even today, graduation day, is no different. I look in the bathroom mirror below my left eye, where *something* brushed my cheek. A lingering sense of genital memory, it's like an invisible and yet indelible birthmark.

✚

I can't quite believe how fast five years of medical school has disappeared. I made friends and relationships, the former lifelong, the latter not so much. The majority of medical students probably don't feel ready to become a doctor. A REAL *doctor.*

Sitting in Elphinstone Hall, off the cobbled streets of old Aberdeen, we are seated ready to collect our degree certificates in alphabetical order. Just months ago we were in fancy dress 'beerienteering' around the city centre, far from looking like soon-to-be doctors. Now we're in fancy dress again, kilts, suits and dresses, about to become *the* most trusted members of society. The Dean calls my name, so I step up to the stage to collect my certificate and look at the applauding crowd, catching my parents proudly, wanly clapping and waving, with the air of people who hope this graduation will be the last.

In medical school, there is always a cushion of not *really* being responsible for anything other than your own learning. Coasting around the wards, trying to absorb information and teaching, sometimes genuinely interested, other times zoning out as hunger hits, or drifting off thinking about student life and 15 per cent discounts. Now, though, there is a terrifying sense of responsibility, that everything we do from tomorrow onwards *matters*. Today the glamour of photo opportunities and social-media posts in full graduation attire. Tomorrow bodily fluids and discharge summaries. We go out into the world as qualified medical practitioners. It's going to be quite a 24-hour jump.

In the UK, your first two years as a doctor are known as the Foundation programme, FY1 and FY2. You spend this time rotating through different medical specialties every four to six months, before you start choosing more specific paths like surgery or GP. It's never guaranteed where in the country you'll go or if indeed you'll get a job. After ranking all available UK posts, you then fight out your application score versus every other final-year student in the entire country, like a massive talent contest.

For our graduation year, the score is based on two substantially different factors. Fifty per cent is made up from your entire medical-school examinations and performance. The other 50 per cent is from the Situational Judgement Test (SJT), a bonkers 'exam' that asks you to rank the order in which you'd react to various situations. Some situations are relevant, but others seem obsessed with asking what you'd do if, for example, you caught a colleague hungover, or having sex in the staff room. With answers that range from 'have a quiet word', to 'speak to your supervisor' or shout 'wa-heeeeey and take photos for the WhatsApp group'. You can't revise for this exam, it's supposedly testing your judgement as a person, something you'd hope medical school would have done *before* gambling five years training you up. With the SJT marks and medical-school ranking added together, whoever is top in the UK has the first pick, then the next and the next, and when it gets down to your score, either your choice will be free or taken.

Luckily, I manage to navigate this process and that results in a job back south of the border, closer to family. Being eight hours away in Aberdeen means I've only seen them sporadically over the last five years, each time amazed how much my nieces and nephew have grown. One time during those five years, I came back badly needing a haircut and shave. I gestured at my hair to my niece.

'Guess what Uncle Ted needs?' (Clearly indicating a haircut.)

'Um. A girlfriend?'

They grow up so quickly.

+

When you think of a doctor, you might imagine a well-dressed person, with a leather case complete with a stethoscope popping out and someone who returns each evening to a nice, homely home. The reality is, my accommodation as a doctor is worse than anything I've experienced before, and I've been camping in March. With a salary and looking to get a place quickly, I take a chance to get myself on the property ladder. The trade-off is moving into a wreck of a place, recently vacated by an elderly lady. Initially I saw it as an adventure, making my own home. Everything inside has been stripped bare apart from the bathroom, which weirdly remains entirely intact, with its convenient hospital-style flooring, complete with shower that is only usable when sitting in the chair. 'We'll throw the bathroom into the deal for you,' the estate agent said, as though it were the deciding factor. Elsewhere, dusty floorboards are all that remain, and indeed I get to know this dust well, as my first few months are spent sleeping on an inflatable mattress. On the morning of my first day as a doctor, I wake to find the mattress has lost the inflatable part of its title, leaving me on the floorboards. I go downstairs and take my seat in the shower, pulling the cord for the water to limply start flowing, splashing onto the dulled green floor. Is this what being old is like? I feel sorry for the elderly lady sat here before me. Covered in soap suds, I start rinsing the house dust away, but the water stops. I pull the cord again, nothing. For ten minutes, covered in soap, I try to get the shower to work, but nothing. Sitting naked, covered in suds, on my first day as a doctor, I realize this shower needs to finish elsewhere. So I pull on pyjama bottoms, jump into my car and drive to my brother's, half-naked, to finish showering. As I arrive, my nieces are coming out the house for school, 'Oh look, Uncle Ted! It's his first day as a doctor!' I gesture hello with urgency and run in topless.

✚

I make it to hospital just in time. I'm struck with how big and foreboding this place is, a metropolis of wards and corridors. Goodness knows what it feels like to patients. I find my way to induction with lots of other fresh doctor faces, pick up an ID badge and then endure a few extremely dull days of fire safety, clinical governance and suchlike. If the military used boredom as an interrogation technique to make criminal suspects crack and release information, it would be based on an NHS hospital induction.

My job *really* starts a couple of days later, and my first placement is on Paediatrics. Anything to do with children is traditionally in a bright and welcoming part of the hospital. Bright colours, decorations, fun posters and toys, stickers and games. A general mix of smells emanates in the ward: hospital, normal life and toast. It's odd that you go from 15–16 years old being on a cheery children's ward, to adult wards that are grey and glib. I join the morning ward round, where Dr Berry, the consultant, is trailed by junior doctors listening and writing what she says in notes or ordering the tests she wants.

One thing you learn from medical school is that hospital is a safe space for letting off any farts. Whereas home life is restricted, in hospital you can get away with gaseous expulsions in the long, wide corridors. Odours blend in with the cacophony of other bodily smells. I am feeling particularly nervous on my first day, plus last night I treated myself to a takeaway. This combination of nerves and spice are fighting in my guts when the ward round reaches a child who has been in for a few days. They are desperate to go home to their video games. I, too, am feeling desperate. Dr Berry is talking to both patient and mum, slowly. I am holding it together and in.

'OK, well, shall we see how things are this afternoon and if everything is settled, we'll let you go?'

I frantically scribble this plan in the notes and sign my name, role and signature, anything to keep my concentration on the page. Focus, Ed, and hold it together. My writing becomes more and more erratic as I fight my bowels. I follow the consultant and other doctors out of the room, giving them a few steps' head start, then while closing the patient's side-room door, I silently relax and feel complete euphoric relief as I uncork my tension, my eyes rolling a little. I start to follow the ward round to the next bay before Dr Berry ahead of me suddenly stops.

'Ah, I left my pen in there, hang on.'

To my horror, she wheels round and heads towards the invisible noxious cloud, which hits her olfactory nerve just as her hand touches the side-room doorhandle.

'Oh . . . my . . . God,' she says; everyone looks concerned, I beam red with embarrassment. She coughs and holds a hand to her face, holding back a gag.

'Ed . . . '

Does she know it's me?

'Ed . . . Ed. My goodness, that *smell*. OK, scrap the afternoon review, no discharge, keep this patient in tonight,' she coughs again.

'Absolutely, Dr Berry,' I say, unflinching.

✚

To say your first year of medicine is where you flex your clinical skills would be an utter lie. A lot of the job as an FY1 doctor is admin, on computer systems that appear no better than a post-zombie apocalypse abandoned office block, where you've managed to reboot the generator and get a dusty screen going. Sometimes a good day or bad day is determined by how long the computer takes to log in while your consultant waits next to you. Anything over three minutes (which is frequent) and there's an exasperated sigh, and you are always made to feel as though it is your fault.

Life is made easier if you know how to quickly order tests, check results, load up X-rays, sweet-talk radiologists into doing that scan your consultant asked for, writing discharge summaries, updating the list for handover and more. You are a glorified secretary to the medical profession. Yet I barely find time to eat or drink. There is no set lunch break, so you have to take it when you can or risk not eating at all. Such is the volume of work some days, I resort to eating a chicken sandwich while hiding in the toilet.

'Finally,' Lucas sighs in exasperation, with more feeling towards me than the computer that took seven minutes to log in. Lucas is a registrar (the nomenclature of doctors is confusing: in short, everything under consultant is 'junior doctor', but registrars are more senior 'junior doctors'). He seems to act like he is already a consultant, with a dry wit and short temper. He certainly seems to make early judgements and I am keen to put across that I'm capable, unlike this NHS IT system.

I started with another new doctor, Alice, who happened to be a graduate like me before heading to medicine. We are both on ward round with Lucas today. Despite having got some of our bearings, everything is difficult to achieve in the timeframes Lucas desires, even the simplest of tasks. Lucas would ask me to fetch something and I'd go off searching, not knowing where to look. It was like working in a supermarket where I didn't know where anything was. 'Finally' greeted me after several expeditions.

'Right, you two,' Lucas points at the patient list, 'this boy currently has chickenpox. I take it you both know your chickenpox status?'

'Yes,' assured Alice, 'I've definitely had it.'

'Great. Ed?'

'Um,' I look around to see if anyone has the answer. 'I don't actually know.'

Lucas rolls his eyeballs. There's something uniquely embarrassing about holding up an entire ward round while everyone watches me call my mum to check if I've had chickenpox.

'Yes! Mum says I've had it.'

'Finally,' Lucas says, opening the door to see the patient.

Life experience is an advantage in medicine. For instance, having children makes you more experienced with common childhood illnesses. I spot this with Alice, who has children and whose learning is accelerating, whereas mine is thwarted in trying to remember even my own childhood ailments.

✚

When I am called to review a young girl on the ward, her parents immediately point out something they have noticed, some heavy swelling behind the nipple. They ask if I know what it is, so I ask for a chaperone and examine said nipple. It is like nothing I've seen before, no skin changes, but sure enough swelling right there, underneath the nipple. No similar swelling on the other side. Was it a blocked gland? I write up my notes, then inform Lucas, keen to make good of myself after the chickenpox incident, and prove I don't need to call my mum to answer every question. My moment of redemption. He joins me to see the patient and has a look.

'Ah yes,' he says. *Finally*, I thought. This will ensure his respect moving forwards. 'This is what's known as a breast bud.'

'A what?' I say, looking blank.

He turns to me with a dry-witted air.

'Often, Ed, children go through this thing. It's called puberty.'

'Puberty,' I repeat cheerily to the parents watching us both.

'Which results in natural changes to the body. A breast bud is one such thing,' he looks to the parents, 'and nothing to be concerned about.'

'Wonderful,' I say.

'Come on, Dr Patrick,' he says, walking away, 'I'm guessing I need to tell you how babies are made.'

✚

A few days later, I start getting to grips with the job, while my home becomes less inhabitable. A plumber has temporarily installed a hose that will rinse me down with lukewarm water, giving me that luxury feeling of prison in my own house. I don't even have to sit in the shower seat for it.

Barely a week in, and it's my first ever night shift. Not only does that mean looking after the children on our ward, but also those on others and any that come through the children's A&E department. We cover a large area of the hospital, just one senior and one very junior doctor (me), with a prehistoric device called a bleep (or pager). We've had smartphones for a while now, but NHS IT is like your stubborn grandad who refuses to move on to new technology.

✚

It only takes one sick child to take your focus away from all the other jobs, and in the winter bronchiolitis, a respiratory illness of youngsters, tends to be the villain. The bleep goes off incessantly all night, seeing such ailments in children down in A&E, while both my registrar and I are spread apart, attending a variety of needs, from being called to the children's cancer ward, to prescribing medication, back to A&E where a child may or may not have drunk some fabric detergent, but the bottle is now empty. What was in it? No one seems to know. The child looks happy and healthy. They're running around the play area shouting 'I'm a train, ZOOOOOOOM!' They don't look particularly unwell, but I don't want to risk it.

'They say it was a clear liquid,' my registrar says, ponderously twizzling the empty detergent bottle in his hands. I look at the brand, then turn to the computer, looking like I'm doing something very serious and technical. In fact, I open up YouTube to look for an advert that might have clues. Aha! There's someone happily filling their washing machine, pouring the liquid in and . . .

'Look, it's a purple liquid!'

'Ah! Great! OK, let's just observe for a bit and if OK they can go home later. Good work, detective.'

Sometimes it doesn't feel like medicine at all.

On my last night shift before a week off, I receive a call to another ward to take some blood tests for a child with cystic fibrosis, a genetic disease that affects various organs, preventing them from working correctly. It disrupts normal organ functions by making mucus much thicker – for example, in the lungs where the mucus is sticky and thicker, thus cleared less easily, which makes the lungs vulnerable to recurrent infection. It's particularly tough on teenagers, who can end up with frequent hospital visits. I knock on the door and say hello to Lewis, who's 14 years old. He has been in for a while, so he's brought various items from home, including his games console that is hooked up to a TV. He's sat on the bed, playing on his phone, wearing a hooded jumper with the hood up. At first, he doesn't say anything. I think he's ignoring me, but when I move closer he looks up and reaches into his blond hair to remove his earphones.

'Blood?' he says knowingly.

I'm not the first doctor he's seen. He knows the routine better than me.

'Shall I put the tourniquet on?' he offers, as I assemble various bits of blood-taking stuff together. I eventually do the honours and we start chatting about football, video games and how hospital sucks because it's boring. I agree.

'First time, I'm impressed!' as he watches the blood being drawn up through the needle. Not squeamish in the slightest. 'Most doctors seem to take a couple of goes.'

'Yes, thankfully I'm better at this than *Fortnite*.'

I write the blood forms and my bleep goes off to see other patients, so I bid Lewis farewell, finding I'm buoyed by our chat.

I spend annual leave catching up on sleep and trying to have some domestic appliances installed, finding the week of freedom flies by quickly as I upgrade my squat living. On my first day back, I'm called to the same ward where I saw Lewis. While there, I see one of the registrars and ask how Lewis is getting on.

'Lewis?' She looks at me confused, then realizes who I'm talking about. 'Oh. Lewis. Sadly, he died last week.'

I stand, feet welded to the ground and mouth open. 'But . . . '

'Yes, it was very sad, he went downhill very quickly. Sorry, got to go.'

She wanders off to see a patient and I am left at the nurses' station, aghast.

I go back to the toilets where I've eaten multiple chicken sandwiches, except this time to digest something else, something more ruinous. I'm distraught. Cystic fibrosis is just a cruel, cruel disease. I start Googling treatments, research, any ideas I could think of to treat it. A futile few minutes, just doing anything that makes me feel more proactive. If this is what I'm like after meeting a patient once, what happens when someone I have cared for longer dies? I look up from my phone. Fuck, I feel fucking sad. I pull hard at the hair on my head until it hurts. I know. 'Come on, Ed,' I say to myself. There are children out there on the ward that need my help. I'll do everything I can each day, but I've got to accept we can't save everyone.

Back home that evening, I arrive to my place flooded with water. I call the plumber – no answer after several attempts. Eventually I call another as I can't sleep in water.

'Sure, I'll be around soon. By the way, which plumber did you have before?'

'It was Luke's Incredible Plumbing Service, LIPS.'

'Ah, ha, Leaky Luke.'

'Leaky Luke?' I repeat, thinking this doesn't sound good.

'Yeah! That's his nickname. Leaky Luke. And you just found out why.'

✚

I learn that in children's medicine, there's a lot of sadness. NAIs or non-accidental injuries are something I become accustomed to. Anything suspicious will be flagged, and immediately safeguarding measures and various enquiries take place to protect the patient. One day, not long after Lewis, I join a consultant and other staff in talking to parents about a potential NAI, a suspicious fracture, in their child. My job is to write everything down. My hand is aching and trembling after two pages, but it goes on for about fifteen pages as the parents and circumstances are quizzed. The parents look terrified and we feel it too. We don't want to leave anything unturned, in case it is the worst case. In case it gets worse. In case something terrible happens to the patient we have a duty to protect.

The scale of children and teenagers attending A&E after intentional overdoses or self-harm is harrowing and, without a question, incredibly traumatic for all those involved. It's not unusual on night shifts to see children turn up after several episodes of self-harm or overdoses, desperate for help. The complex nature and lack of time we have to assess them and ensure they are fit 'enough' doesn't allow you to fully get into the history of the problem, or indeed anywhere near solving it. By the time you start to scratch the surface, the bleep goes off, calling you to emergencies and jobs across the other side of the hospital. We admit, refer to the mental-health team who will see them in the morning and then discharge. I'm so sad and frustrated at seeing young people in need of help, taking overdoses or cutting themselves, yet we can only offer limited support in and out of hospital. It's not by choice that we don't step in and up. We have no faculty to do so, nor time. And the worst part is that these abuse and mental-health issues go unnoticed right until an emergency hospital attendance, where the resource-stricken NHS struggles hard to provide safety and support.

✚

Over the next few months, I become more adept, learning the permutations of paediatrics. Everything is smaller: the needles, the blood-collecting bottles, the medication doses. You become a master inquisitioner of nappy contents, looking for problems with feeding or dehydration. How many full nappies? What consistency? Colour? You start ignoring the bewildered look of parents at your questioning. You appreciate the power of play assistants in distracting children so that you can examine them, and you become highly skilled in the blowing of bubbles to win crying children over. Rapport is the key, and you do anything silly to build it.

In adult medicine there's an unwritten rule of pleasantries. Generally, hellos are exchanged and questions of 'what can I do for you?' are answered accordingly. But children will tell you how it is and that might range from laughing to crying, or to unannounced vomiting all over your shirt.

✚

On entering a room to examine a child, I am greeted by screaming. It could be because of my face, but hopefully it's not personal and he just hates hospitals. Listening to the heart and lungs is nigh on impossible in a screaming child, so I look for clues to calm the situation. I spot Spider-Man slippers.

'Oooh, look at those *awesome* slippers! Is Spider-Man your favourite superhero?'

'No,' comes the retort, the tears ceasing a little.

'Well, who's your favourite?'

'Lightning McQueen,' he says with such seriousness that the crying stops to fully engage in this important discussion. I have no idea who Lightning McQueen is, so enquire further.

'He's this amazingly super-cool car.'

After a few minutes of talking through Lightning McQueen's attributes, I try my chances.

'Shall we do a superhero check-up? Like Lightening McQueen would have?'

Glee replaces crying as I substitute medical examinations for an MOT.

'Let's hear how the engine sounds' (I listen to the heart) 'and now the exhaust' (the lungs) 'and let's look at the wing mirrors' (ears) 'and the rear-view mirror' (throat).

I am getting through it all as the father is sat reading a paper. Lucas knocks on the door and enters to find both me and the boy making car sounds and laughing.

He looks to the father.

'Which one's yours again?'

Lucas is dragging me out as there's a child needing a lumbar puncture (also known as a spinal tap), where a needle is placed into the back to obtain some fluid that surrounds your brain, to check for meningitis in this case. It's something I haven't done before, so he assists while letting me do the procedure. The young boy gets into position on his side with the aid of his parents. Not only am I successful, but when the results come back it shows zero red blood cells, known in the profession as a 'champagne tap'. I gleefully inform Lucas of my success, especially as rumour has it that the tradition is to buy the doctor a bottle of champagne.

'Nice try, Ed. However, you do get your name engraved on the trophy.'

Lucas reaches up to a dusty, paper-laden shelf and brings down a plastic pot with a Lego man bent double on the top, with a spinal needle hub stuck into its back. A white sticky label is attached with a name and a date from last year.

'Look at that, the first one for over a year!'

Lucas scribbles the date and my name on, then returns the trophy to its dusty, out-of-sight home.

Just as I feel I'm starting to get good at the job – my few months' rotation is soon to end – still every day I seem to see something new. My bleep goes off to take some blood down in A&E. I can't even see the veins, let alone stab one. Savini, one of the more energetic registrars, excitedly offers to help. She's so friendly and full of energy that I think she'd explode if she ever downs an energy drink. She joins me in the room with our two-year-old patient, mum and dad.

'Ahaaaa! Little one has no veins to play then?' She bends down and beams a smile at the toddler who smiles back.

'Luckily I've brought my magical tool.'

I hope she's not referring to me.

She whips out of her pocket a bicycle torch, switches it on and to everyone's surprise turns off the lights. We're in complete darkness aside from the torch she swings around like an emergency lighthouse. While she is wildly gesticulating in the darkness and swinging the light around, I'm blinded several times, then it goes dark again. I cannot see a thing. I stumble to my left and bump into mum and dad

'Sorry, sorry,' I say, like I'm getting to my seat in the cinema. Savini has found the toddler's hand and has placed the torch underneath it, so that the light shines through the skin, causing it to glow red and highlighting some blood vessels.

'Ooooooh,' from both the child and Savini.

I decide to sit down before falling, slowly lowering myself into a chair and appreciating just how comfortable furniture in the children's department is.

'Ed, can you pass me the needle?' Savini asks. *Absolutely not* is my first thought. I can't see a thing. Everyone will end up with a needlestick injury if I play this version of pin the tail on the donkey.

'I need the light on, Savini . . .'

The light flickers on and I discover my comfortable chair is actually an extremely shocked dad. I'm sitting in his lap.

After my final shift, I move on to a new placement, so a brief celebratory drink in the pub and then we're gone. New doctors will arrive on the children's ward and all we've done here will be forgotten. Not me, though. I got my name on the champagne-tap trophy on a dusty, forgotten shelf.

Chapter 3

It is the end of my first year fully qualified and I'm finally feeling more accustomed to being a doctor. And this time I am off to A&E.

But first my passport is due for renewal, and I'm excited to add the title 'Dr' onto it. All the hard work, exams, money spent and training gives me this little perk at least. Off I go to the passport office with my degree certificate and information, and excitedly ask the nonplussed passport officer looking at my form.

'I'm a doctor now, too. Can that go on my passport?'

'Yes, no problem,' he says unimpressed, not looking away from the paperwork.

'Great, so I've got all my evidence and ID here . . . ' I start rummaging through my bag excitedly.

'Nah, no, it's OK, I believe you,' waves away the officer.

Wait, what? I thought.

WHAT?

Five years in medical school grinding out for *this* moment, and anyone can just walk in and *ask* for it? No checks. No proof needed. I'm damn well showing him my degree. I get all my ID and doctor paperwork out and place it on top of the form he was reading. He looks up at me, like I'm an idiot.

'Yeah, man . . . I said no problem.'

'I just wanted to show you all of it, all of the reasons I am a doctor.'

✚

Contrary to the glitzy celebrity doctors I've seen on social media and TV shows, with chiselled looks and snazzy hospital settings, perks and glamour are nowhere to be seen as I look up at the jaded A&E sign and entrance, my hair askew from the pouring rain. Exhaust fumes blast in my face from cars and ambulances, while the doorway is busy with people moving in and out, some pushing wheelchairs and others in arm slings.

Dripping, I find the office where I check in for my first shift, a tiny side room off the main corridor to A&E, where other doctors starting their A&E rotation queue out the door for special green scrubs, so special that we have to pay a deposit for them. I am grudgingly allowed three pairs instead of two, when I point out a

15-day run of shifts I have coming up means I'll either be coming in scrubs still wet from washing or full of BO. The secretary hands me the third pair and takes another £20: £60 deposit right there. I'm so glad I could use that prize money from medical school for this.

My confidence in hospital has grown as helping acutely unwell people becomes more routine and I am especially looking forward to A&E since *any* type of medical condition can come through the door. I very much hope that this will give me insight into what I most enjoy and therefore *what* path of medical training I should take. Hand severed by knife, perhaps it is surgery I was destined for? A woman giving birth in my hands, maybe an obstetrician? Hiding in dark rooms to escape? Perhaps I'll be a radiologist.

✚

Every area of the A&E is a bit grim. There are a few side rooms with doors that serve as the fanciest offerings, but most beds are in bays, close together, separated by only curtains. Some days this would be sufficient, but on others even a small increase in demand suddenly sees the department full and spilling over. We're seeing patients in corridors, without adequate privacy. Maybe we should have medical school exams where we see patients in busy corridors: it would be much more realistic.

In the bays, it also means everything is audible: every bodily function and malfunction, as well as conversations. I feel this lack of privacy when I see Ronald, a man in his 70s who has had a fall. As I walk into the bay, there's an energy to his smile despite feeling under the weather. He already has an IV drip going into his arm, but he's otherwise relaxed. His shoes slightly muddy from some gardening, he wears a woollen Rotary Club jumper with the sleeves rolled up and there's a general musty smell of sheds. He's got all his faculties about him, but he's hard of hearing and shouts his replies, meaning our conversation takes time and is pretty much broadcast to the rest of the hospital, as well as in A&E. Our consultation is convoluted. When I introduce myself as Dr Patrick, he thinks I'm offering him a taxi. When I ask about any allergies, he says cricket isn't really his thing. With some charade acting skills, I manage to get through most of my questions sensibly, then begin to look through his list of medications and there's one I don't recognize. I could go and look the drug up, but as I'm with Ronald I ask him what it's for.

'It's for the old soldier, doc,' Ronald says.

He's not heard me.

'Yes, but what is this medicine *for*?' I say, trying to animate for communication again. 'This SIL-DEN-A-FIL,' I say loudly in syllables. Miming suggestions of headache or backache.

'I told you, for the old soldier,' he replies, matching my volume.

'But what is the old . . . '

I stop as Ronald begins to gesture to his groin.

Before I can communicate my cognition, Ronald bellows so loud the whole department hears.

'It's to get me cock hard, doc!'

A chorus of laughter breaks out from behind every curtain in the bay.

'Yer know? I call it Viagra. Here, when me and the wife . . . '

'Yes Yes Yes,' I say, hoping he'll stop.

'I can tell you more about it?'

'*No*, that's quite all right,' I say.

'You can have one if you like, you look a bit deflated.'

'No, Ronald.' I can hear everyone laughing again. 'But thank you.'

Ronald is cheerily smiling, and the rest of the bay is settling down from hysterics. I come out from behind the curtain to find doctors and nurses have surreptitiously congregated to hear our conversation play out and I also notice the wheezing of two laughing asthmatics has got worse.

A&E also means the end of having any semblance of a social life. Previous jobs had some element of regularity where I could occasionally see some friends or family, but A&E shifts start and finish at random. No one else seems to have lives that revolve around working from 15:00–24:00 or 20:00–05:00, sometimes for 13 days in a row, especially not when it comes to dating.

Carlos was the registrar on today. Some registrars are excitable and have bundles of energy, some are quiet, some are stealthy and difficult to find. But Carlos is friendly and famous for always wanting to know 'what the bloods show'. Even when a patient didn't need any bloods, that would still be his first question. I'm pretty sure he doesn't listen and asks anyway. He notices me as I sit next to him on the computers, exasperated as I look at my phone.

'What's up, Ed?'

My social life is spilling into work time and I look at Carlos, unsure whether to disclose my dating shenanigans.

'Ahh, I dunno, just someone I'm dating.'

'Go on, tell me, I'll help you, pal,' he says still looking at the screen.

He *is* always friendly and it's not like I've got time to discuss it outside these hot and sticky walls.

'Well,' I start 'we've been on a few dates. It's fun but we live *so* far apart, plus these shifts mean we only see each other after night shifts. I just don't know where it's going or what to do?'

'OK,' he turns to me with all seriousness, 'and what do the bloods show?'

✚

Other A&E colleagues and I make up for not having lives outside by sharing anything unrelated to medicine.

'Look, Ed, look!' Sarah, one of the other second-year doctors sidles up to a table where I'm making some notes. Sarah, an avid animal lover, regularly shows pictures of her and friends' animals during the brief moments of pause between major incidents.

'How *gorgeous* is this little doggy?'

I 'oooh' and smile, envious that I have no canine friend, but also aware I don't have time, or a home fit for humans yet, let alone dogs.

'You know, Sarah, you'd make a great vet?'

Sarah shakes her head and screws up her face.

'Me? Oh, no no NO. I couldn't do it. I'd be far too sad if any *animals* died. Right, which patient shall I see next?'

She grabs the notes from the 'to see' pile and wanders off. I wish her next patient all the best.

✚

If you've ever been to A&E, you'll know there are generally two entrances, ambulances at the back for very unwell patients, or the front for those able to walk in. Patients attending A&E either come into hospital to stay, or go home. It's slightly unnerving deciding whether to discharge someone home, as generally it's the first and only time you ever see them, so I end up panicking that all my patients will burst into flames and die once they pass through the exit. Whereas a GP has the luxury of booking a follow-up appointment, someone turning up to A&E is a snapshot moment, where you're under pressure to find out if there's a real problem and sort it out as quickly as possible if it is life-threatening. You can spend hours doing blood tests and investigations, believing that some medical mischief is at large, only for all those tests to come back normal and the patient can go home. On the flip side, everything can *seem* normal and then you find out it's not.

✚

Natasha is only five, so has been brought in by her parents rather than attending alone. I walk into the waiting room and call her name. This is always a good indication to see how sick a child is. Natasha comes, bouncing off the walls, excited and giggling, carrying a teddy, while her parents are grateful and apologetic for their not-so-sick looking child. They're worried because they think she might have swallowed something. They're not sure what, they were just in a room together and heard her cough. Natasha hasn't been ill or complaining of anything, but they have a gut instinct something is up. I'm currently watching her run around the A&E playroom, at full pelt, laughing and smiling. Examination and observations are completely normal; it seems appropriate to reassure and discharge. I screw up my nose, thinking something does seem *odd*. I order an X-ray, something that you don't do lightly in children as you try to limit radiation exposure, but the story was strange and the parents are concerned. The X-ray comes back and I load it up on the computer.

'Oh shit!' I exclaim at the doctors' station. Everyone comes to look.

'Oh shit!' people say in unison.

Sitting in Natasha's lung, lodged at a perfect angle, was something like a spring, to a pen maybe?

'Aha, I was wondering why my clicky pen wasn't working,' says the mother.

I make the necessary referrals and vow to *always* trust my instincts in the future.

+

At around 01:00 that night, aside from a couple of drunk injuries, the A&E waiting room is for once not rammed. The hot and sticky air that fills the department when it's full has lifted a little, and the registrar has said I can go on a break. I wander to the coffee machine to find it is out of order, then the vending machine for a can, also out of order. Another vending machine for food has a solitary, tragic potato in a foil parcel that for *just* £3 will be all yours. I almost buy it out of charity to set it free. Instead, I head to the staff room to find nourishment options there. In the small box room I find some teabags, and after thoroughly cleaning one of the mugs dunk it in there with some hot water and milk to boot. There are no spoons, though, so I clean off a knife that has been used for cake earlier, withdraw the teabag and finally enjoy my tea. I sit down on an old sofa and my tiredness lets me imagine what it would be like if operating theatres were stocked as well as staff rooms.

'Scalpel, please.'

'Sorry, we're out of scalpels. Can I interest you in a spoon?'

+

The night shift starts to get busy. My tiredness and hunger pains increase deep into the morning. Luckily, I strike biscuit gold when a nurse in the children's part of A&E shows me the secret bourbon biscuit store.

'Here, Ed, don't tell anyone,' she whispers, opening a tucked-away cupboard to reveal stacks of bourbons, and my stomach makes a deep thunderous sound. The bourbons are technically meant for patients, but as a doctor, restricting children's sugar intake feels responsible. I ponder this while putting an entire, unbroken, chocolate bourbon in my mouth. Once I've managed to swallow it without choking, relieved to have finally eaten something, I go to see seven-year-old Jimmy, who his parents have brought in because he has a lot of pain in his groin. A nurse chaperones as I examine the painful area that is his testicle. I'm pretty sure this is testicular torsion (simply, the testicle twists inside the scrotum, cutting off the blood supply). Just the thought of it brings a tear to the eye (of most people with testicles). As it's 08:00, I ask Dr Taylor, one of the consultants, who's just arrived to start shift, to come take a look.

'Certainly is torsion, we'll need the surgeons. Just make a diagram in the notes showing which testicle is affected, Ed.'

Despite being exhausted, I open the child's notes and set out the sketch, my final task before bed. I realize after half a page has been taken up that I've never drawn this sort of thing medically, only on my desk at school. I look down at the cartoon line illustration of a large erect penis I have just drawn in a child's medical notes and panic and cross it out. I draw a much smaller more medical one on the next page.

'Oh my goodness!' sighs one of the nurses at seeing the tarnished official medical notes. She points angrily at the page.

'Honestly.'

I brace myself for a telling-off.

'Some of the children coming into *this* department, drawing obscenities over medical notes! They need a good telling-off, I tell you.'

I nod in agreement and wander off, a bourbon in hand, as I grab my things and head for the exit.

✚

The self-discovery of finding out the things I like and dislike isn't quite as existential as I had hoped. But I do discover I don't like doing rectal exams (AKA putting a finger up someone's bum). I abhor all the aspects to it – from the jelly-like lube, right up to the gloved warmth of someone's anus. The medical term for this examination is PR (per rectum), so there's always a childish giggle among doctors when they meet someone who works in PR. I can't explain why, and although I've still not 'found' my medical specialty, I most definitely don't want to work with any arseholes (which I guess rules out orthopaedic surgery too).

Which makes me think what doctor would *enjoy* doing it? My aversion means my heart sinks when I know it needs to happen. I glaze over as Mrs Shaw, telling me her problems, has now given me plenty of reasons to perform said examination. Some abdominal pain, her bowels not opening for a few days, blood on last time of wiping. Not doing a PR would be negligent. Who'd have thought you could get into trouble for *not* putting a finger in a stranger's rectum?

I explain it's a test we need to do and she's quite understanding.

I get things ready and find a nurse to chaperone, then take a second to psychologically prepare myself. It's not my first rodeo and I've had enough experience with this that I know that the more confident the practitioner (or PR-Actioner), the more comfortable the patient is.

So, I snap on some gloves in what I hope appears a confident fashion (thinking to myself, I may fear the anus, but at least I respect it).

'It's quick, a bit uncomfortable, but won't last too long,' I explain.

I get Mrs Shaw in the right position, lying on her side, knees up to chest. We're out of lube in the room, so I ask the nurse if they know where to find some, and they pop off, returning a few minutes later.

'Here you go, doctor, let me squeeze some on for you.'

'Yes, lots, please.' *Always* be over-generous with lube in any PR examination. I lift a buttock to inspect the anus for any problems while lube is squirted onto my finger. Looking like a painter sizing up the canvas while holding his paint brush away, I smooth lube around my finger to ensure full coverage ready for insertion.

Strangely, it becomes more difficult to move my fingers.

I try and rectify this by amping up the pace of my movement but eventually my fingers stop moving. I look back at my fingers, they're all completely stuck together.

'There's something wrong with the lube,' I say to the nurse.

'*Lube*? Oh, I thought you wanted glue?'

At the word 'glue' I notice first Mrs Shaw's anus and, then, my own, clench.

'Glue? Why . . . would I want *glue* for a rectal exam?'

Realizing I was seconds away from being attached to my anatomical nemesis, there's a period of silence as we wait for the real lube to arrive.

'Sorry about that,' I say to a concerned-looking Mrs Shaw.

'No problem, I don't want you sticking *to* my bum, that's all.'

'You're not alone, Mrs Shaw . . . '

✚

You can tell what time of year it is by what comes through the A&E doors. On Halloween, I X-ray someone dressed as a skeleton, which is surprisingly satisfying. Christmas and New Year bring in tinsel and increased drunken injuries. Valentine's Day brings in romance and . . .

'You fell on it?'

I try *not* to raise my eyebrows in disbelief.

'Yeah, just, you know, slipped off the sofa and . . . and . . . '

'Your trousers fell down and the remote control ended up lodged there?'

'Yeah, exactly! Sort of . . . '

'No problem, I'll have a chat with the surgeons right now.'

Whatever the story, the treatment is the same, extraction of foreign body from the rectum.

I move to open the side-room door.

'Ooh, doc. Could you ask the surgeons to save it for me? I don't have another remote and, well, it accidentally logged me out of Netflix on the way in.'

Irrespective of the season, our job in damage (remote) control remains the same.

✚

Our role in among the A&E chaos isn't always straightforward. We're drilled to see patients, diagnose, treat, admit or discharge, repeat. Sometimes there isn't much we can do medically, and I feel powerless with James, who comes into A&E with his partner. He has advanced, inoperable cancer, has been through multiple rounds of chemotherapy and all treatments have been explored. He's been given the devastating news recently that nothing more can be done, he's dying. He's come to A&E because there's more abdominal discomfort than usual, but the main issue is that they're scared of what will happen, scared of dying. Who could blame them? They tell me they just didn't know where else to go.

The routine tests and investigations show nothing has changed. His blood results are off the charts, as expected. His liver is massive, as I feel the rugged edge of it beneath yellow, jaundiced skin. In A&E there's generally always something you can do or at least try, but I feel helpless.

I feel fucking sad, sitting at the computer staring at the blood results I can do nothing about. What if it was you? Maybe there is something I can do. I call the medical team and speak to the registrar on call.

'Look, I know there isn't a clear reason to admit this patient, but I don't know what else we can do. They don't feel safe anywhere, we can't just discharge him.'

'No, we can't. Let's bring them in overnight and see what we can do.'

James and his partner are grateful and clearly comforted by the news. I'm just one doctor they see fleetingly on this awful journey and I feel helpless in their plight, but at least it's something. There's a wait for being transferred to the ward, so I keep checking on him, to see if he's OK, until I see a porter pushing his bed out the doors, which swing shut, and he disappears.

✚

It's a busy shift and one of the nurses is trying to look after a drunk patient, who keeps shouting her name at regular intervals. All of us have gone in to explain that 'No, we're not a bar' and 'No, we can't bring alcohol into the hospital'. Despite our pleading, that it's late and other patients are being disturbed, he continues to shout after the nurse, Delilah.

'DELILLLAH' echoes around the department.

It becomes apparent that the intervals of shouting happen at surprisingly regular intervals and I notice one of the other drunk patients starting to count down, while signalling to the other drunker patients around them.

On cue, they all start singing.

'My, my, my'

'DEL-LIL-LAAAH!'

'Why why why'

'. . . DEELLIIILAAAH!'

In such perfect harmony that it makes all of us, including Delilah, brighten up.

✚

There's no stopping in A&E. On to the next patient, then the next and the next and the next and the next. They never stop pouring in. The busy days where the department is rammed full, where ambulances queue up outside and corridors become wards, go fast, leaving me shattered. The slower-paced days drag, feel longer and also leave me shattered. My snacking has increased a hundredfold, my sleep pattern has been broken into pieces of three-or-so hour intervals (no matter the time of day) and I miss having more weekends off.

When the end of my A&E rotation comes, I turn up to the same office where we collected the scrubs from. There's now another queue of doctors waiting to get their special greens, ready for A&E. I pop ahead of the queue just to drop my scrubs off and collect my deposit.

'Oh, just keep them,' the secretary waves me away.

'I thought we got the deposit back for returning them?'

'Yes, but sadly someone has stolen all the deposit money, so consider it a parting gift.'

A parting gift, three new pairs of pyjamas.

Chapter 4

My final ever Foundation Year job leads me to freedom. Being outside the hospital.

No nights, no working weekends unless I choose to. What is this *sorcery* they call *General Practice*?

✚

Working in GP is a privilege in other ways too. I'm out of hospital, in the real world. I can pop out to get lunch, do home visits, even have my own room to work in – with a door, no less. Away with those pesky curtains. I now have things that indicate a person is about to enter my threshold. The other privilege is being a doctor working in arguably the most recognizable health job in the public eye. Almost everyone has seen a GP or at least knows what they do. They are the front of house of the NHS, the link from primary to secondary care. No longer would I be awkwardly walking into bays to see patients. They would be coming into my room. I would greet them with a swivel of my computer chair, stand up and offer them a seat. There might even be plants, greenery or art.

How civilized.

How very grown-up.

✚

On my first day at the practice, I stand outside the building in raptures at what lies ahead of me. I have already discovered that I can park for *free*, and there are plenty of wide spaces too. I shake my head in disbelief and look for hiding ticket inspectors or signs, but it's genuinely *free* NHS staff parking. Is this heaven? Have I reached NHS nirvana?

I peer up to look at the practice – I'm no stranger to how buildings fluctuate between being nicely modern and absolutely decrepit. By my luck, this was the latter. I tilt my head at the flat-roofed eyesore, noticing a patch of grass beside it desperately trying to plaster on some sort of natural feeling. Still, it's what's inside that counts, I ponder, as I gaze back at the car park.

'Ed, is it?'

I switch my focus from the building to where the Scottish lilt has come from and find a man with a briefcase just locking his car.

'Yes, are you Dr McNeal?'

'That's me all right. Call me Hamish.'

Hamish is one of the GPs in residence and he is also assigned to the role of my supervisor. He joins me at the building and peers up at it.

'A beauty, isn't it?' he says dryly. 'Just wait until you see inside.'

Inside, the corridor and rooms are a comfortable marriage with the exterior. The dated carpet has edges curling up and silver gaffer tape covers cracks in both the walls and floor. All the staff greet Hamish with a cheeriness that seems over-exuberant given the health and safety trap they operate within. Hamish introduces me to the four other GPs that work in the practice, each varying their greeting. Dr Khan is extremely smart, with stylish hair and a wide smile. He gives me a firm, bone-crunching handshake and I manage to keep smiling despite the pain of his enthusiastic welcome. Dr Adam contrasts this with giving me a loose, wet handshake. Literally wet: he apologizes as he's just washed his hands. I hope so, wiping my hand dry on my shirt. Dr McBride, seeing my hand get the Dr Adam treatment, offers a little wave while sipping a coffee. She's the longest-serving GP here, but tells me her real passion is making jewellery out of placentas. Just as my face starts to contort, Hamish leads me off on a tour.

'Yes, I know. Weird. So, as you can tell, we're a mixture of GPs,' he says, escorting me into what I can only believe must be the kitchen as there is a kettle. He reaches up to get some teabags and cups before continuing.

'Everyone has their own style. I admit the place is a shithole, but a functional one. By that I mean this thing,' he points in the vague direction of the kettle. 'This works and so do the toilets.' He stops and flicks the kettle a couple of times until the light on the side comes on.

'Everything else is a little unpredictable. Except the printers. These are the damn finest printers the NHS has: you click print and they print.'

We both acknowledge this basic yet rare NHS attribute, as we move out of the kitchen and he affectionately taps the printer in passing.

'So you'll get your own list and just ask if you need any help. You will also do house visits and you can join me today. Sorry, do you want a tea?'

After a morning of shadowing Hamish, which largely consists of sitting in the corner of his examination room looking like a scolded child who has been told not to speak to all patients who enter, he then informs me that we are off to visit a nursing home. His car is strewn with paperwork and a child seat is covered in crumbs at the back. He puts his arm behind my headrest and reverses out the space.

'Just cross fingers we don't get stuck behind an old person.'

We're not long on the road before we're stuck behind an elderly driver in a slow-moving yellow car. The road gets more and more windy and countrified at each corner.

'Every. Time.' He shakes his head and mutters.

'Honestly, *every* time I come out on visits, the elderly population joins in to stop *me*, a doctor, seeing other elderly people . . . Wait, wait, maybe that's it? Maybe it's all a conspiracy by the bowls club members to kill off their rivals?'

We come to a stop at traffic lights and Hamish, slightly flushed, opens the window to cool down a little. When the light changes to green, the yellow car crawls at a painfully slow pace, such that we nearly miss the light changing again. Hamish, now red-faced with frustration, grips the steering wheel with white knuckles and does an impression of someone accelerating a car while not in gear.

'BrrrrrrrRRRRRRRRRRRRRRRRRRRRRRrrrrr . . .

'EVERY.

'TIME.

'I tell you.'

Our trip to the nursing home is followed by a few house visits. Medication and patient reviews, checking any minor complaints and answering concerns are the main orders of the day. One thing becomes all too clear. Hamish the GP is treated like a local celebrity. People are *very* excited to see the doctor and he laps it up while introducing me as his sidekick. Less consistent are the places we visit, ranging from homes that are meticulously tidy to smoke-filled and porcelain-figurine-cluttered.

✚

Things don't seem any different at the practice. Without having my own room to see patients, I am shovelled into whichever GP's room is free each day. I am a sort of migrating, rudderless doctor. The rooms themselves vary massively in states; some are clean and tidy and some have multitudes of old coffee cups and plates strewn over the desk, or paperwork jostling up against family photos. One GP's room seems to be that of a hoarder, with old egg cartons, pots and jars with mould, and all sorts of countryside trinkets littering every surface. I wipe my hands across the desk, trying to quickly clear it up before a patient enters, and when I sit down in my swively seat I see black dust across the palm of my hand. Without fail, a set of weighing scales is in each GP room, used every day by me before I see the first patient.

✚

On one of the busiest days I have encountered so far, I am ushered into the only room I've not yet had to pretend is my own and clearly the least used out of the lot. It's unclear why. The frosted window is on the right side of the building for natural light. It's spacious too. I notice files with the name of a doctor I've not met on the top shelf.

'Who's that, then?' I say to Shelley the receptionist.

Shelley looks up, frowns, looks at me, then moves a chair to stand on and turn the files around, hiding the name.

'Well, you can Google it if you like.'

I Google and find that said name on files no longer works there, or likely anywhere, after being caught having sex with a patient in this very room. I look around and feel a bit nauseous. It was a long time ago and the room is relatively tidy compared to the others. Still, I grab some wet wipes and spend thirty minutes cleaning down everything, paying special attention to the bed. Afterwards,

I sit in the soft reclining chair. This is *very* comfortable. I suddenly jump up to clean it too.

✚

It is on this day that Doug, a 40-something builder with a crowd of tattoos decorating his upper arms, has come to see me, complaining of abdominal pain. He's now feeling nauseous too, but given that he doesn't know the history of this room, I'm guessing it's because he's unwell. Paint and dust cover his overalls as he's come straight from work after not being able to eat his lunch. It's the first time we've met, but he's clearly in severe discomfort, so we cut to the problem, pain.

'It's just been getting worse, doc.'

I get him on the freshly anti-bac'ed couch and examine his abdomen. To touch, he's tender on the right lower side, a clear indication that this could be his appendix.

'I think we need the surgeons to have a look at you.'

I call the hospital and the surgical registrar asks for him to head up there. In A&E it would be a referral and that's all I'd hear of it, no follow-up or anything, but in GP you do. A couple of days later, I call Doug to follow up.

'Oh, hi, doc, you were right, appendix. They said it was

inflamed so took it out and let me go home yesterday. Got a few days off now, thanks very much.'

Wow. HOW satisfying. Not just diagnosing and referring, but being able to follow up too, having the full picture from initial prognosis to outcome.

'Doug, that's amazing. I'm so happy for you!' I realize it sounds like I'm congratulating him on giving birth.

'Yeah, sure, doc . . . No big deal.'

As I put down the phone, Hamish knocks on my door and pops his head in

'Do you want to watch a big cyst being removed?'

Before I gather my thoughts on whether or not I truly do, I'm in the treatment room where Hamish is doing some minor surgery. Mr Rushcliffe, his 79-year-old patient, has a large cyst on his scalp but is happily chatting away about a waterpark trip with his family as Hamish injects local anaesthetic.

'My grandchildren *insisted* that I join them on this slide. I was reading the paper and tried explaining that Grandma said I wasn't allowed, but my wife overheard me fibbing, so off I went.'

Hamish makes an incision, then starts to squeeze. Clearly, Mr Rushcliffe is oblivious to his scalp being sliced open, and on he goes.

'And this slide, it had so many twists and turns that I was feeling dizzy, the kids were screaming and loving it, then before you know it – SPLASH!'

At the word 'splash' the cyst pops everywhere. I manage to hold off vomiting everywhere too.

'*Very* satisfying,' says Hamish, smiling at his work.

'Absolutely,' says Mr Rushcliffe. 'I think the impact must have doused everyone at the poolside.' I gingerly check my face hasn't been too.

✛

I begin to learn that GP life is where office work and medicine meet. Lots of leaning on doorways and chatting, with biscuits. A whole mixture of paperwork, patients, practice staff and copious amounts of tea. Which is very quintessentially English but has begun to play havoc with my anti-diuretic hormone (ADH). ADH is a hormone that prevents water from leaving through your kidneys, which means that the tea makes me pee a lot. To begin with, I try to be as discreet as possible about this increased urgency, but when we are rolling through patients every ten minutes I have to make quick jolts for the toilet when the chance arises. It gets to the stage that if one of my patients cancels late in the day, the receptionist, Shelley, fills the booking system appointment with 'Dr Ed's pee break'.

✚

I find being a GP freeing. You are your own boss, have your own patient list and work independently from anyone else. Every time I am doing house visits it feels like an escape, mixing with the real world rather than going from one ward to the next. As the temperature climbs up to a heatwave in summer, the sun bakes the practice building, so going out into the car for blasts of fresh air is a delight. In hospital I'd be melting. If I finish house visits with time to spare, I visit a local woodland for lunch, lie down on some grass and stare up through the trees while shovelling cheese crisps into my mouth. It is bucolic. I would never be able to do this in a hospital car park.

✚

The day-to-day becomes routine, from people with coughs and colds, aches and pains, skin problems, to mental-health troubles, with some hay fever here, some high blood pressure there, although I realize pretty quickly that the prerequisite ten minutes is never enough for the majority of patient appointments. People come in with one problem, but have lots more they want to talk about, a little like going to the shop for flour but then thinking *well, I might as well get my weeks' worth of food while I am here.* Some issues just take longer to discuss in order to find the root of the problem. Sometimes, though, a little reassurance is all that's needed.

Jake is 44, with greying hair that flows onto his T-shirt. He has found something in his mouth. No symptoms, nothing is giving him problems, but he's seen these things happen before and they're apparently not right.

'OK. Let me have a look,' I say, grabbing a pen torch and wooden spatula to press down his tongue. I look at the back of his mouth and throat, pink and glistening with saliva, but I can't see anything unusual.

'It all looks absolutely fine.'

'You can't miss them!' he says. 'There's two massive dangly things at the sides, at the back.'

I look again, confident now that the offending appendages he's referring to are tonsils.

'They're your tonsils, perfectly normal,' I reassure him.

'They weren't there before.'

'Before when?'

'Before I looked.'

After a bit more toing and froing, we pause and I realize we're at a stalemate of discussion. We need an independent adjudicator to settle this, so I ask Hamish, who agrees to look only *after* I convince him in front of reception staff that yes, I *do* know what tonsils look like. We both pop back in.

'Yes, they are your tonsils,' Hamish asserts.

'OK, thanks, phew, I was worried I might die tonight,' Jake exclaims.

Finally, we've managed to reassure him.

'No no,' Hamish says. 'I'm pretty sure you'll make it until the morning.'

✚

Occasionally, it's me that comes across as unbelievable.

'Olive oil? You want me to put olive oil in my ears?'

Emma, in her 20s, is holding back her long, dark brown, curly hair to reveal her ears. Her problems lie further inside as she has come to see me about some ear-wax difficulty, and olive oil is a treatment option. You can buy it over the counter, but most people have some in the house, so why waste the money?

'Just a few drops,' I say.

'But I cook with that and put it in salads?'

'Oh yes, I wouldn't cook with it after.'

Emma stares at me, clearly wondering if I've gone mad.

'Honestly, try it and I'll give you a call to see how you're getting on.'

I print off an information leaflet, to give my treatment some credibility, but Emma clearly wonders if I've just typed it up and added an NHS logo. She laughs and takes the leaflet, then wanders out the door shaking her car keys.

Thinking my next patient might believe me more, I welcome James into my room with a smooth chair swivel, my best yet. Even James, in his 50s, who is sporting a deep tan and is wearing, to my horror, a full-on winter jacket in this heat, seems impressed by my glide from sitting to standing to greet him.

He's been bitten by an insect and the surrounding skin around the bite mark has become erythematous (a fancy way of saying very red) and hot. It's a skin infection, so I prescribe antibiotics and also pull out my pen from a drawer.

'Shall we draw?' I suggest.

'I . . . I'm just here for the appointment really.'

'I mean on your leg.'

'Again, I'm just here for . . . Oh, is there a reason for it?'

'To check the antibiotics are working. If the redness goes

beyond the line, you'll need to go to hospital.'

'I guess you . . . should draw then.'

After drawing on James' leg, he looks bewildered and leaves the room. As it's my last patient for the day, I stretch with a celebratory yawn, put my hands on my hips and stand on the weighing scales. The sedentary lifestyle of a GP is adding to my paunch. I open the door and see down the corridor James is speaking animatedly to Hamish and showing him his ankle. Hamish spots me.

'So, Dr Patrick has been drawing on you, you say? *Highly* unusual. Maybe he's Banksy and you're his latest canvas?'

'Well, yes. That's what *I* was thinking. Maybe you should have a word?'

'Absolutely, he could at least make the lines join up.'

It is still peak summer and I am a seasoned GP at this point when Hamish asks me, 'Do you want to work this Saturday? Admittedly for free, but it's fun.'

I raise my eyebrows at the combination of working for 'free' and 'fun'. Hamish covers local sports events, and there's a long-distance race where doctors are needed at stations. Despite my cynicism, it does actually sound fun.

We arrive at the midway station and have a small tent for people to come in with any niggles or ailments. At the beginning, it's mainly elite athletes passing through, none of them stopping at all. This is *easy* work. Hamish tells me it's later, when less experienced 'athletes' come through, that things get going. Sure enough, a few hours into the event a trickle, and then a flood, of people come to the medical tent. All of them with foot blisters from rubbing trainers or socks. I spend the entire morning either popping blisters or taping padding onto and around them. Manky sweaty foot after manky sweaty foot depositing blister fluid is proffered in my direction. The further into the event, the worse the feet become. At one point I can't tell if my hands are sweaty or just covered in blister fluid. When the people dressed as charity mascots come through, it gets worse. 'You are *kidding* me?'

Hamish laughs at my disgust as I remove the trainer and sock of a participant dressed as a dinosaur. For a second, I think their wrinkly, reptilian-esque foot is part of the costume, until a blister bursts in my hand.

✚

My time as a GP begins to near an end, just as I've started to master parts of it. I've got the tea-making skills down, I know the computer systems and enough local town and traffic knowledge to seamlessly break the ice with patients.

As I wait for my next patient, I look out the window and think how great it is to have weekends off medicine, unless you're into dinosaur's feet. But it comes with a stark awakening: I *miss* the hospital too. After just two years of being a doctor, I now have to choose which specialty to work in if I want to continue training. But I'm exhausted from rotating, and undecided. Although I will probably look back at these months with envy and awe if I move back into the strip-light world of hospital care, the pace is a bit too slow for me here, with the only thing fast-paced being my trips to the loo.

✚

It is around this point in my reverie when I notice that a young and healthy woman called Jessica is in my room. Having come from an exercise class, she wears sports leggings and a hoody, with bright purple running shoes. She tells me that she has come to see me with some pain and swelling in her arm. I think to myself that it all seems pretty straightforward. She explains that it is starting to bother her a bit, despite taking painkillers. We get chatting, as she's applying to university soon and isn't sure what to do.

'Who is?' I say knowingly, actively refraining from telling her my life story.

She mentions that she has started going to the gym recently, so I reckon this is a case of muscle tenderness, maybe pulling or tearing it after exercise? But as we chat, it becomes clear she hasn't been doing any arm exercise. I examine her arms and notice a slight swelling on the one giving her bother. Strange. I pop in to one of the GPs and ask their opinion. They suggest booking an ultrasound scan.

'Let's book an ultrasound scan,' I say, returning. Then I have another thought. I leave GP soon and an NHS ultrasound will be around six weeks, that's if we're *lucky*.

'And an X-ray too,' I add, just to be sure. 'You can get that tomorrow at the hospital.'

Jessica thanks me and leaves with a bounce.

The next day, I get a call from Shelley saying a radiologist from the hospital is on the phone.

Agh, they're going to scald me for booking that ultrasound scan. I cough and pick up the phone.

'Hi, it's Dr Patrick here. Is this about the ultrasound scan? I can explain.'

'What? Oh no, nothing to do with that,' the radiologist

says, surprised. 'I've just reviewed your X-ray. It's highly likely osteosarcoma.'

'What?'

I almost drop the phone, and my mouth hangs open.

Cancer of the bone.

✚

I speak to Hamish and we organize Jessica's regular GP to join me in a follow-up appointment to break the bad news. I call Jessica to come back, to bring a family member with her if she can. There's a horrible silence that echoes when you break bad news, every syllable reverberates around the room from the shock of each word being said.

Confusion,

disbelief,

tears.

All hang between us.

In the space of a few short days, I've met Jessica and delivered devastating news. I feel sick and guilty. People commend me for the fast diagnosis, but I don't want to talk about it. My rotation finishes soon, so I won't even know what happens. None of my remaining appointments feel the same. I still think about the fortuitous booking of an X-ray. If we had waited for the ultrasound, it would've been so much longer: the delay for referral and treatment, the impact on Jessica, her family, her future. It sits heavily on me and I take some of the shock into my last few days as a GP.

✚

You and I, we all forget that ultimately doctors are the same as patients. We are all veins, heartbeat, blood, emotions. It can seem we're made of stronger, more resilient stuff, and indeed perhaps it's more palatable or even therapeutic to think your doctor is confident and right in everything, as that way they are more godly and less human. In truth, we can be just as unsure or insecure as the next patient in the waiting room. We check our phone too much, we eat unhealthy things, we drink, we develop bad habits, we worry about friendships, relationships, family, money, the future and whether we're doing the right job both for us and for our patients. It can take one traumatic experience, a patient dying in front of you, an error on your part, a toxic work environment that makes someone leave a job, or medicine altogether. It's luck what situation you walk into. And sometimes bad luck can destroy you.

✚

After my last day the following week, Hamish takes me to the local pub for a send-off. He asks what I'm going to specialize in and I try to do my best to articulate with shrugs and head shakes.

Hamish interprets my explanation and takes a deep breath.

'Listen, at the end of the day it's a job. You've got to live a life outside of it, otherwise it swallows you up and spits you out and it doesn't care what it does to you. I chose GP because it gives me a freedom. A freedom to choose how much I work and when I work. I don't want to work nights, or in a hospital. It's great.

'But don't get me wrong, there's some crap. The paperwork is endless, the resources are stretched, we can't give all the appointments patients need, you finish late mainly because of admin, admin, bloody admin. It can take a toll on family life. Some GPs sub-specialize only so they don't have to do pure GP all week, because it's exhausting and draining. On top of that there's the paperwork, hoop-jumping festival of appraisals, all thanks to Harold Shipman. The best thing? It's the patients, it's *always* the patients. Sure, I do events so I can have a break, get outside and occasionally get free entry to festivals. Do something that lets *you* live outside of work.'

With that grand monologue, it is my time to leave medical training behind.

And try and find out what I should be.

Chapter 5

It's not the end of medicine for me.

How brazen would that be? A doctor writes a book and five chapters in *quits* medicine altogether. Does he retreat to a simple life away from civilization, living in a cabin among mountains and rivers while herding cattle?

'What the fuck am I going to do?' Alice says, wiping away tears. 'I *still* haven't got a job here, I don't know what the fuck I'm going to do.'

On our way back from some locum shifts in hospital, I was trying and failing to console Alice, with whom I shared my first doctor job on paediatrics. She applied for surgical training but hasn't got a job offer anywhere near where she lives, meaning she can't take it. Otherwise, her husband has to quit his job, her children have to move school and they have to sell their house.

'Well,' I start, trying to find something positive, 'you can do whatever you like for a year then try again?'

'No, no. I need it *now*. I'm not like you, I *want* a structure to my life. I've got kids, Ed, I can't just fuck about.'

I have a potted plant to worry about, but decide this might not square up to Alice's two-plus children. I do want structure. Trouble is, I just don't know *what* structure that is yet.

You would be forgiven for thinking that doctors seamlessly continue through training to becoming a consultant; that having completed medical school, everything becomes a much smoother, stress-free process. And guess what, it's the opposite.

The deeper you get into a career as a doctor, the more nuanced the problems of job applications become. Everyone knows that to become a doctor you need to get into and finish medical school, assuming after that, hey presto, you're a doctor. But afterwards come the trials of getting different jobs in different specialties and the outcome of success varies wildly. One thing is ubiquitous: you rarely get much of a say as to *where* you get your job; it's more hope and luck. So, for people with families and children, that's pretty important. For those with a single potted plant, like me, less so.

I have chosen to enter the no man's land of medicine. No training programme, no supervisors, no support system, no job. It is freedom. Freedom or unemployment, depending on your perspective. The unofficial 'FY3' is a doctor's gap year. The medical wilderness, whereby doctors in the UK work their first two years (FY1 and FY2), get to the point of applying for a specialty, but for a variety of reasons don't and drop out. They're not GPs or surgeons or anything particular, they're junior doctors just like me, in limbo either by choice or bad luck. It wasn't the plan medical overlords had: the idea was for doctors to head straight from FY2 into specialty training. But the toll of being a junior doctor takes hold, with burnout, wanting flexibility, to travel, try new experiences, work in other sectors or abroad, buff up the CV, earn more money or see friends and family more often. There's also indecision over the different careers. There are more than ninety different medical specialties, and you only get to work in four to six of them during the first two years as a doctor, after which you're expected to pick your entire path. In 2010, 83 per cent of FY2 doctors entered specialty training, whereas in 2019 only around 35 per cent did. Some come back to medicine, but others never do. They vanish into the non-medic world.

Even without this, there's such a shortage of doctors in the UK that gaps in rotas need filling almost everywhere you look, meaning locums (ad-hoc shift fillers) are constantly needed. Most doctors in training experience these shortages, with rota gaps a roulette of being filled and unfilled, some days well staffed, others not so. You end up working exactly the same shifts alongside someone else who is paid three or four times as much as you. By filling locums it means junior doctors can do exactly the same work but are paid much better, plus have the flexibility of choosing when to work. This isn't unique to doctors – nurses, midwives and more all have the same issue. Until rotas are staffed adequately and people are paid better, no amount of publicity or government statements of 'we've got x number of extra doctors' hides the fact that there are huge NHS shortages. If there weren't massive rota gaps, locums wouldn't exist.

✛

For me, I don't know what kind of doctor I want to be, plus I want to see more of my family and friends, take a holiday and get some more experiences. Taking advantage of my freedom from a medical rota and the potential to work something resembling sociable hours, I apply for a teaching job in a medical school.

The interview for the teaching is informal, a walk around the medical school while two professors suss me out. The school looks like a barn conversion, an old building that's had an uplift. Exposed brick and wooden beams go alongside models of skeletons and classrooms. It feels odd walking around a medical school as a doctor now, the worry over taking assessments or exams shifts to the idea of marking them instead.

✚

Teaching brings new surprises, and seeing it from the other side as a doctor, I know what is expected or needed in hospital. Not so much in medical school.

'Foreskins?' I raise my eyebrows and check I have heard correctly. I was helping Peter, a fellow colleague, set up for catheter training this afternoon.

'Yeah, there's a bag somewhere if you can find them in the store cupboard. They're fake,' Peter strains while putting out a model penis, *sans* foreskin.

'Well, I'm glad you said store cupboard, I was about to go to the anatomy department and see what I could dissect.'

I wander to the back of the medical school, passing a hubbub of students and other academics, looking for a bag of foreskins.

I find said store cupboard and, lo and behold, a bag of fake foreskins, sitting there in a clearly felt-tip-labelled box in among the stationery.

Walking back, I nonchalantly toss the bag from one hand to the other on my way, when I run into the Dean of the medical school, who is showing some official-looking people around. He suddenly accosts me for a PR moment (not that kind).

'Ah, Ed, come, come. Now, Ed here *is* a doctor, who's a clinical educator, teaching the students today, well regarded and knowledgeable. What's that you've got there, Ed?'

He smiles, looking for me to continue the good impression. I start to hide the bag a little more.

'Oh, it's nothing.'

'Well, come on, what is it?'

I reluctantly and slowly bring the bag out in full view of the important-looking people, who squint.

'It's a bag of foreskins.'

'A ... bag of ... foreskins, *Ed*?'

'Yes, I mean, they're not mine,' I add.

'Why are you carrying ... '

'Good question, so they're for the catheter models. You slip these onto the ... the ... '

For some unknown reason, the word 'penis' disappears from my brain. I search for alternatives in the nanosecond I have and nearly start gesturing but manage to abstain. The silence is growing, I have to say something, *anything*.

'Willies. They're for the catheter willies. I don't know why you have to buy the foreskins separately, that's not what happens in real life, is it?'

The professor smiles and ushers the guests away from me quickly, as they look back to the rubber skins. I look in the bag and count ten foreskins. Who needs *ten* foreskins?

In the afternoon, medical students attend the clinical-skills session and I'm given female catheterization to teach, complete with an anatomical model, which thankfully does not need any foreskins. Lancelot, a particularly posh and slightly overconfident medical student, comes to have a practice.

'Have you seen one of these before?' I gesture to the model vagina.

'Yes. I've had a couple of girlfriends and . . .'

'Ah, no, Lance, I mean specifically this model. Have you used the model before?'

He looks at me, perplexed.

'To put in catheters?' I add.

'Oh, sorry! I thought . . . No, I haven't. But I can do catheters, no problem at all. Very confident.'

I'm not sure if his confidence is misplaced, considering he thought I was asking if he's ever fornicated with the medical model. I quiz him about the process for catheterization before deciding how much teaching he needs.

'What kind of water do we use to inflate the catheter balloon?'

I'm looking for the answer 'sterile', but I'd accept 'clean'.

'Oooooooooohhh.'

He looks at me, thinking hard. The blood vessels on his temples engorge under the strain.

'Still?' he offers.

My eyes widen in surprise, but he looks nonplussed, happy with his answer. I just love that *sparkling* was his other option.

'Let's start from the basics then.'

✚

I keep searching for medical experiences, so book onto an outdoors medicine course – several days of learning how to Ben Fogle or Ray Mears yourself out of tricky situations by purifying water, skinning rabbits, tying knots and building shelters. While also caring for someone injured on a mountainside. The endgame on the final day was a medical scenario set in remote woodland, where someone had fallen off a cliff. Our job was to extricate them to a safe point for the helicopter to collect. There are eight of us in our group, a mixture of paramedics, nurses and doctors. We all hike out excitedly to the woodland, crunching sticks and leaves beneath our feet and seeking the map point where our severely injured actor is waiting and snacking – right until they see us, that is, when they suddenly start making mouth-filled sounds of pain –

'Awwwwowwwawww!' Then they go back to snacking while our instructor details the scenario we face.

After stabilizing them as best we can, we set about making a stretcher out of sticks and clothes, and the patient is transferred onto it, still snacking away on grapes as we work around them. As we start to lift the heavy stretcher, we now appreciate there are eight of us, yet wish there were more. Slowly we move through woodland, with over two miles still to go – *Jeez, this is tough*. I try and peek at how the others are faring and whether they might want to take a short snacking break. But then the instructor shouts, 'The patient is now in cardiac arrest!' We slowly drop the actor and simulate cardiopulmonary resuscitation (CPR) until the instructor says the heart is working again. We start moving again, two minutes later 'arrest!' and the same thing happens. It continues on and off and there's an audible sigh from everyone, including the actor, as they're dropped to the ground with an increasing thud each time. On about the sixth arrest, an anaesthetist in our group sighs and holds her hands up.

'Guys, they're dead.'

We all look up, puzzled, as we catch our breath.

'Look, we're in a hilly forest, and we keep moving and stopping to do CPR, but they're arresting each time we move because we didn't figure out the problem as to *why* they're arresting. We have no equipment to do anything else. Whatever we missed, we missed at the start. So, they're dead. *Dead* dead. They're not going to survive arresting every couple of minutes while we carry them a couple more miles through this terrain.'

We look at each other, reluctantly agreeing with the summary, although our sadness at failing the simulated scenario is offset by not having to carry the snacking actor, who is even more displeased at having to walk back.

✚

I suppose to myself that I could drift along, teaching and working shifts, but I don't think that is where my work satisfaction truly lies. I want that medical structure, to get back to training. I just need to figure out *what*. I book up all my annual leave and buy a plane ticket to New Zealand, to meet up with a friend, Billy from medical school, who had also left UK training like me, opting for more exotic climes.

At the airport for departure, I take this first opportunity to use the title change on my shiny new passport.

'I don't suppose you need a *doctor* in business class?'

'No, we don't. Here's your economy boarding pass, *Doctor* Patrick.' The check-in clerk hands me the pass and smiles with a glowing please-fuck-off-ery.

Sitting on the plane to Auckland, I take a pen and start processing my thoughts. Some people know exactly which specialty they want to do from medical school, or even from birth, it seems. They carve out impressive CVs in preparation for interviews, while many others still find their way. It's enviable that some people are so set and can plan. For many, like me, it's more a case of ruling things out until finding one that fits. I scribble 'surgery' on a piece of scrap paper and immediately cross it out. I like being in operating theatres, but surgery is not for me. I can barely carve out a Sunday roast, let alone an appendix. I go through my past jobs. In GP I missed the urgency and I sat down too much, whereas I like the immediacy, the urgency and emergency of A&E, but missed the follow-up time with patients. In paediatrics, I enjoyed working with children, but missed caring for older clients too. All of them crossed out, my field was narrowing. I consider others like haematology, infectious diseases and microbiology, but none of it gives me the excitement like parasites, and there's only a small scope for tropical diseases in the UK.

On my paper, as it has been in my head, one specialty stands out as I circle it continuously. Not for the first time either. I've answered questionnaires designed to match you to a specialty and this has popped up several times. I've even attended career-guiding seminars that pointed me there, too. It's always been mooted as a specialty that would suit me, even friends suggesting I should do it.

Anaesthetics.

Throughout my time as a doctor, I've only seen an anaesthetist if there was an emergency, when someone can't breathe or is severely unwell. Each time, the anaesthetist would float in, calm and unconcerned by the commotion. There's always a sigh of relief. Each time, I was slightly in awe.

My first anaesthetics encounter was on medical-school placement in Inverness. I was offered coffee and, assuming it would be the watery hospital stuff, I declined, only to then be shown into the staff room where, taking up most of the surface, was a barista coffee machine with two espresso ports and a milk frother. I thought they'd stolen it from Costa. I was impressed.

Aside from the coffee, there's one other thing that stands out for me in anaesthetics: time.

Time with a patient or even to yourself is something you rarely get enough of in parts of modern medicine. I've seen busy medical registrars in hospital departments sit down and suddenly be swarmed by people asking different questions about different patients, all while their bleep goes off with calls to other parts of the hospital. But in anaesthetics it *has* to be one patient at a time, your sole focus on the person in front of you undergoing an anaesthetic, and being with them throughout the operation through to recovery. This could mean minutes or hours with the same patient. Mention this luxury to doctors working in a specialty like A&E and their mouths drop open a little, their eyes widen. I swear some even drool.

Before we take off, I start looking up applications and check the Royal College of Anaesthetists website. Their coat of arms is populated by golden morphine poppy heads and cocaine leaves, more the kind of crest you'd expect for a drug cartel than medicine.

I start thinking about my own anaesthetic experience, having only ever had one general anaesthetic. I clearly remember the moment of going under. I was nine years old and told to count backwards from ten, but when I got to seven, the drugs and gases took hold of my brain, I looked up at the anaesthetist and said 'Wow, you look like a right plonker.' There was a pause, the sound of laughter from nurses, the stony, unimpressed face of the anaesthetist, then I was out. I always wonder what happened after that moment. Either way, I'm glad to have woken up.

However, the most powerful anaesthetic I experienced as a child was when Dad accidentally shut my hand in the car door. The pain was unbearable and tears rolled. Dad quickly offered me £1 to not tell Mum and stop crying before she came back to the car. The thought of sweets made the pain disappear instantly.

✚

After the long flight, I arrive to find Billy, complete with sunglasses and surf shorts, having just finished night shifts and got an hour's surfing in before meeting me. He's opted for surgery and is staying out in New Zealand 'forever', he says. I tell him about my thoughts of becoming an anaesthetist.

'Ah, yes! You'd be perfect! Plus you can work with me and do all the important stuff I need, like press the button to make the operating table go up and down.'

✚

I'm torn because I love working for the NHS but also realize how poorly staff are treated and paid, and contrast this to the time Billy is having. But the thing bringing me back to the UK, like many others, is family. Just before I came out to New Zealand, Dad became ill again, requiring more life-saving surgery. Moving abroad, so far away from my family, would mean constantly living in the shadowlands of fear and worry: worry about receiving a phone call with bad news and not being close. Nor do I want to be far from my siblings and their families either. Before I take the plane home, I decide to apply for anaesthetics, NHS style.

✚

On arrival back in the UK, there's a delay to leaving the plane. The tannoy comes on.

'Ladies and gentlemen, we're sorry to inform you there's a delay due to a man in the airport terminal, possibly with a weapon.'

No more details are known. Not knowing what will happen (it turns out to be a false alarm), I worry, think of my family and emotionally text Mum.

'Mum, there's a man in the terminal with a weapon, I don't know what will happen but I love you x'

Mum replies.

'OK, hope you're not delayed for too long.'

Chapter 6

'**Shit, shit, shit!**'

I was in my anaesthetics interview, part of which consisted of walking into a room and finding a question on the table with a pen and a large piece of paper.

'How are doctors different from other professions?'

I had ten minutes, now nine minutes, to write, then deliver a presentation to some consultants sat next door. Where to start?

Six minutes.

I pace the room.

I look out the window and see a football ground. I grab the piece of paper and start drawing a football stadium, then players, photographers, ticket sellers. Then I add a high street and different shops.

Three minutes.

Whatever I'm doing, I can't go back now, this is it. This is the summation of everything I have worked towards. My medical career aspirations rest on whether I can sell this poorly conceived urban landscape. Is this an anaesthetics or estate-agent interview?

One minute.

SHHHHHHHIITTTTTT.

The buzzer goes, and a door opens, seemingly by magic, leading into a room with anaesthetic consultants in. There is an expectant atmosphere.

'Hello, Dr Patrick, if you'd like to present.'

I pin up my paper and take a slight cough in the silence, aware of how my drawing skills are no better than when I was six years old.

'So, this is a football stadium and high street.'

Some surprised looks.

I persevere, explaining that footballers are role models like doctors, but more to entertain; these are the photographers who want to take the best shot – 'As do the strikers,' I add for some light pun activity.

No smiles are offered.

I move on to the high street. 'Here we have a florist that's wanting you to have the best flowers for when you get married, but good luck to any doctor for getting your wedding day off a medical rota.'

Again nothing.

I go through the rest of it in a blur, describing the difference between doctors and other professions.

Poker faces all round.

'Thank you, you may leave.'

What was that?

Whatever it was, it was enough. Soon after, a letter arrives, I am accepted onto anaesthetics training.

I jump in joy and call my family with the news, then double-check the letter is from the anaesthetics recruitment office and not Foxtons.

✚

I hand my notice in at the medical school I'm teaching at and ready myself for a career as an anaesthetist. Let me explain what anaesthetics is. Because unless you've worked with, or ever needed, an anaesthetist, then you might not know what we do. I know this from countless conversations where I assumed people knew, only for it to end 'So is that some kind of doctor?' Often in a fearful 'Is that legal?' way. Indeed it is, and I had finally embarked on specializing as a doctor.

We anaesthetists are somewhat of a medical specialty that was born out of surgeons struggling to do their job when patients were awake or moving, or most likely both. Situations without anaesthetic are a favourite for movies, where someone needs an amputation or a bullet/arrow removing, only to be comforted by something to bite down on and a swig of rum. Since then, we've developed various drugs and gases in what has essentially been a clinical trial, running over several centuries, which has taken many names but should really be called 'what works without potentially killing you'. We still don't have the perfect anaesthetic drug and we still don't know how a lot of them work, but we're pretty certain they are more effective than Captain Morgan.

What drugs did these doctors find that didn't kill you, I hear you ask? Well, let me tell you about three of the types of drugs anaesthetists use.

✚

Firstly, there's the anaesthetic. Chloroform on a piece of rag has evolved into more palatable gases that are inhaled, but we also use drugs injected into the vein. The most common of these is propofol. This is a white milky emulsion that looks exactly like milk, which is useful to distinguish it from other drugs, except a latte. I'm pretty sure you could froth it and not tell the difference. You might be thinking where have you heard the name propofol before? It's probably from the death of Michael Jackson who, via his dodgy physician, was found to be acquiring industrial amounts of propofol plus other drugs, that likely stopped him breathing.

✚

Secondly, there's pain relief. Anaesthetists are experts in pain and making it go away, and we commonly use opiates. Morphine you've probably heard of, but there's stronger stuff too. Diamorphine has got the street name heroin, yet it's exactly what we inject into spinal anaesthetics for Caesarean sections. Then there are the fentanyls, an incredibly potent range at the centre of an opiate crisis in the US, where people die rapidly because they stop breathing or choke on their own vomit. Straight-up fentanyl is what we mostly use, but there's a multitude of others, some too dangerous for humans. For example, carfentanyl is used in animals bigger than cars – good for rhinos, pretty fatal to people. This was seen in 2002 when Chechen rebels held 800 people hostage in a Moscow theatre. Russian troops allegedly released a gas with carfentanyl into the theatre, in the hope of bringing down the curtain on the rebels. It did, but it also killed 120 hostages.

✚

Finally, with more exotic origins, are muscle relaxants, or paralysing drugs. These emerged from curare, a poison used on arrows by Indigenous peoples of South America to catch animals. They'd paralyse the animal and stop it breathing. This was witnessed by eccentric Englishman Charles Waterton, no doubt in full white safari outfit with hat, moustache and a pipe to boot. After managing to obtain some curare, the Yorkshireman brought it back to the UK to perform what sounded like a morbid circus show for his local town. He had three donkeys – he injected Donkey 1 with curare; it fell over and died. For Donkey 2, he wrapped a tourniquet around its leg, injected curare below the tourniquet and Donkey 2 was fine! Then he released the tourniquet and Donkey 2 died. Donkey 3, who was shitting himself at this point, was injected with curare and, by some incredible means, mechanically ventilated (yes, the donkey was ventilated) by Waterton. After a while, the drug wore off and Donkey 3 recovered, living a full and happy life with a couple less friends. The demonstration was so famous that Donkey 3 was immortalized by a mention in the local paper.

✚

Despite the drugs we use being some of the most powerful in health care, there's always a patient information leaflet inside their packets. It always amuses me reading through them. Even the muscle relaxants have a 'Please consult your doctor before taking this medication' and other advice on how to take them. Who exactly is paralysing *themselves*?

✚

There is a darker side to this line of work, as it's a profession that can have grave consequences when things go wrong. As such, we anaesthetists are at a much higher risk of substance abuse and suicide rates are high – the belief being that an anaesthetist rarely fails in their suicide attempt. These drugs have also been used as murder weapons. Jealous lovers have tried to cover up deaths by injecting muscle relaxants and burning the house down, only for the pathology reports to show no carbon monoxide in the body, meaning breathing stopped well before the burning, and toxicology doing the rest.

In 2006 in the UK, a male A&E nurse was found guilty of murdering two patients and harming fifteen others after the hospital noticed an unusual number of respiratory arrests (where people suddenly stop breathing). When he was arrested at work, he was found to have a syringe of muscle relaxant in his pocket, something he should never have been in possession of.

✚

So why am I telling you all this gore? Well, all three types of drug I've described have something in common: they can each and together stop you breathing. So, as well as a glorified (and hopefully qualified) drug dispenser, an anaesthetist's main job is managing a patient's airway and breathing, which often involves putting a tube in the throat and using a ventilator to do the breathing for you and us – because the alternative is for us to squeeze a bag manually to keep you breathing, which would become very tiresome. (Although that is what medical students did for polio victims 24 hours a day in the 1950s, back when they didn't even have smartphones.)

✚

Before I even start anaesthetics, I'm in love with it. Why? Because of the powerful drugs, cool machines and coffee.

My excitement isn't punctured as I grin myself through yet another dry hospital induction. A world-weary IT specialist sets the scene for the day.

'The computer program we use is called Millennium,' he says in monotone. 'Robbie Williams had a song of the same name in 1998, so that tells you how up to date we are.'

I walk around the hospital during the break to get a feel for the place. The smell and laminate flooring have that all too familiar NHS feel, as does the canteen serving up insipid and under-seasoned delights. Nothing seems more typical of an NHS canteen than a sign sitting on a bowl of fruit that reads '30p per piece'. On the same sign underneath it says 'SPECIAL OFFER – 3 pieces for 90p!!'

There were more quirks here than my previous hospital. 'Don't enter this corridor!' hung a sign chained to double doors blocked by two bins and a warning sign. I stare for a few minutes, wondering if zombies are beyond.

'It's condemned,' hushed a porter to me in passing.

'Condemned by whom?' I shout to the porter after.

He raises his arms in a shrug as he walks away. I look back to the chained doors, then back to the porter, who has disappeared into thin air.

After induction we have resuscitation training in a tiny room that I thought was actually a storage room, due to the number of mannequins shoved in it, like the back room of a department store. I have to move a few to get near to the one that needs resuscitating.

✚

My first few months are spent getting to grips with this new specialty. In a way, anaesthetics is the antithesis of what up until now I have been taught to do. To actively make someone unconscious is generally met with panic and General Medical Council referrals in most other clinical scenarios. So, when you start anaesthetics, it's a whole new beginning, with different rules for success. A patient paralysed, unconscious and not breathing for themselves? Superb work, doctor, provided you're doing the breathing for them.

There's also a variety of accepted techniques and drugs, so every anaesthetist becomes individual and develops their own potions. You spend a day with one consultant learning the way they do things, then find someone else the next day does it completely differently. Like a chef, picking and choosing their ingredients for their favoured recipe and method. Sprinkle a few quirks here, some Gordon Ramsay narcissistic tendencies there, and *voilà*, *bon appé*-fucking-*tit*. This means that there's more than one way to do things, one anaesthetist will differ invariably from the next and both are correct. Hopefully . . .

✚

Just as important as anaesthetists (if not more) are the ODPs (operating department practitioners), specialized nurses who assist every case needing an anaesthetic. They are the true unsung heroes: no good anaesthetic happens without an ODP. Taylor is the ODP with us today, and at my every turn of needing something she's there holding it, anticipating everything.

'I'm going to leave the next one to you,' Sally, my consultant, says, finishing her coffee.

'It's for a gallbladder removal. Patient is fit and well, call if you have any problems. All right, byeee.'

A shot of adrenaline runs through me, I've not anaesthetized a patient alone. I've been having fun all this time with the bicycle stabilizers of a senior with me and now . . .

. . . I was being given a *real* go at it alone.

Anaesthetizing is a bit like playing the game where you lean backwards and trust someone to catch you. You allow yourself to be unconscious and trust someone else to make sure you breathe, and for the first time now that someone else was me. And only me. I thought to myself, I'll never forget this moment or this patient.

And if it goes well, they won't remember me.

Drugs are drawn up, everything is ready, so we wait in the small anaesthetic room for the patient to arrive. It is quiet except for the air system that howls through the room from the operating theatre, making it seem like an escape-room game that's about to start. Terence arrives, a middle-aged man who is much more relaxed than me. I greet him and decide not to announce that he's my first ever solo anaesthetic, thinking it might affect his blood-pressure readings. So, instead, I busy myself as Taylor does her checks and I apply a tourniquet to the left arm. A big bouncy vein pops up.

'Delicious,' I say to myself, although a little too audibly as Terence frowns. In goes the cannula. Part one done. I position Terence and hold the oxygen mask over his mouth.

'OK, a few deep breaths, then I'm going to give you the sleepy stuff and we'll see you after the operation.'

I hadn't intended 'sleepy stuff' to sound quite as layman. Hopefully Terence still thinks I'm a qualified doctor and not a nursery teacher. I inject the anaesthetic and after a few seconds his eyes shut and he becomes unconscious, so I take the mask and hold it over his mouth, lifting his chin.

'Can you open your eyes?' I say suspiciously, as part of me wonders if patients fake being unconscious, as it happens so quickly. The monitor then starts beeping to tell me he isn't breathing, so I decide this isn't an elaborate ruse. We wait for the anaesthetic drugs to fully work, which seems like an age.

'OK,' I say, after checking the clock.

'Let's go for it.'

Taylor hands me the laryngoscope, a large metal blade used to help find the trachea. Terence's mouth limps open and I slide it in, all the way back, seeing all the fillings on his teeth and his tonsils and uvula covered in saliva. I spot the dark hole I'm aiming for and Taylor hands me the breathing tube. In it goes. I connect it up and give the bag a squeeze. Terence's chest rises, the tube mists with expiration, I look at the monitor and see a wave in the end tidal CO_2, all this telling me the breathing tube was in the right place.

'Yes!'

Sally enters the room, eating an apple.

'How did it go?'

'Great!' I reply. 'He's not dead.'

'Not yet. How about you turn the ventilator on?'

✚

I find all the surgery mind-boggling too. On monitors I watch gallbladder after gallbladder being taken out, by being put into a little bag inside the patient and then pulled through the small hole in the skin the surgeon makes. Each time, it reminds me to do my laundry back home.

Every type of surgery has different anaesthetic learning points. Sally teaches me during rectal surgery how vagal nerve stimulation by stretching of the anus can potentially lead to the heart slowing or even stopping.

'Wow, there must be people who shove stuff up their ass and just die, then?'

'Yes, Ed.' A pause as the whole operating theatre reflects on my slightly too loud and excited question.

'Interesting first thought,' Sally whispers.

✚

Dr Commons is an anaesthetic consultant I try my best to get along with, although on days I'm anaesthetizing with him he seems unimpressed with whatever I do. Any missed cannula or difficulty putting the breathing tube in is met with derision, he quizzes me on topics I know nothing about in front of patients to make me look foolish, he even criticizes my packed lunch for looking a bit downmarket.

One day, he drifts off topic and suddenly opens up to me, talking about his past relationship. I try to appear considerate and interested. After all, this might be the moment where we finally find common ground and start to get along.

'I loved Julian.' He shakes his head in nostalgic fashion. 'Back in the day, there was a *lot* of sex with Julian.'

'Julian?' I say, still surprised at this honest conversation.

'Yes, right here in this very room. Then Julian had to go.' He looks wistfully across the floor.

'So did someone catch you?'

'What?' he looks confused.

'Did someone catch you? Having sex with Julian, in here?'

He now looks at me in disbelief.

'SUX! SUX, Ed!' he bellows as his face turns crimson.

I also go red at realizing what he's referring to.

'Suxamethonium is a muscle relaxant, Ed. *Julian* is an old style of ventilator.'

✚

Not that it's all popping tubes in. During the on-call shifts we also have to be involved with critically ill patients. Sometimes this ends with them passing away. I fill out a death certificate for an elderly man. Later, Dr Commons calls me.

'It looks like there's a problem with your death certificate. They apparently aren't dead.'

'What?' I say in shock, struggling to work out what he means.

'Because you've certified your *own* death.'

Turns out I put my name in the wrong box.

'The coroner has asked me to check if you are braindead. I said I'd try to find out.'

✚

After a while, I start mentally taking home some work traits. The beeping of monitors is too similar to the beeping at checkout scanners in supermarkets, or parking sensors in cars. Even the anaesthetic assessments we do stay in my mind as I look at other people's faces outside hospital. Things like neck size and movement, how wide someone's mouth can open, or their Mallampati score.*

These all add up when you are trying to predict how difficult it will be to keep someone breathing (and therefore alive) after giving the anaesthetic. At barbecues or other social events, I now can't help but zone out of small talk, look at a person's face and think how easy

The Mallampati score was devised by an Indian doctor of the same name in the 1980s. It gives an indication as to how difficult intubation might be. If we can see all of your dangly uvula and soft palate, that's generally a good sign (score 1). If all we see is tongue and the top of your mouth, it might be tricky (score 4).

or difficult it would be to ventilate them. Even on dates, I wonder how well I could keep them alive if we were stranded somewhere and they couldn't breathe. Oh, look, they're laughing at my joke and I can see their uvula, Mallampati score 1.

✚

Dr Commons always dresses well to see patients and is disappointed that other people don't follow his example. Whereas most anaesthetists in the hospital change into blue scrubs before seeing patients having an operation that day, he sees patients in his smart waistcoat and tie combo before changing, tutting loudly at all the anaesthetists not in the same attire. Adding to his own self-importance, he likes to put on classical music when patients are in the anaesthetic room, to help create a relaxed atmosphere. He takes pleasure in asking me what the piece is called and then revealing the answer as I fail to recognize it. Today, though, I know it.

'Do you know this piece, Ed?'

'Pachelbel's Canon?'

'Correct! Maybe we'll get some culture into you after all. Is it a favourite of yours?'

'No, I've just heard it at every funeral I've been to.'

Dr Commons scowls at me.

Taylor chokes her laugh away as I look down at the floor.

✚

I'm on the way to the eighth floor of the hospital. I say 'on my way'. I'm actually waiting for a lift in the main lobby along with some relatives, porters and nurses. There are eight lifts but only two are in service, because even elevators have workforce gaps. They're like the gateway to the real part of this hospital, as the main concourse is flanked by the commercial likes of Marks and Spencer and Pret A Manger, adding some high-street atmosphere to the infirm. Never before has seeing a sick relative while enjoying a miso soup been so easy.

I'm off to do a pre-operative assessment of a patient, which is generally the first time someone meets an anaesthetist. For everyone having an operation, there are three parts of the journey to unconsciousness. Where you are at the start, the journey to operating theatres and arrival in the anaesthetic room. You see the anaesthetist at the first and third stage, but you're unlikely to see them on the journey unless your starting point is in intensive care. For everyone else, the starting point is a waiting room, a day-surgery unit or on a hospital ward like here.

The pre-op assessment involves seeing and examining the patient, while also doing some detective work in the medical history and notes. We check blood tests, scans and other investigations while also making sure there aren't any surprises that might affect the anaesthetic (it's not unusual to find some medical issue no one has mentioned). One of the major parts is the focused examination, which involves some unusual tests. How many finger breadths can you open your mouth to? Can you protrude your bottom jaw? Can you put your chin on your chest? After doing several of these, I see patients starting to doubt that I'm really an anaesthetist and just some guy who's walked into hospital for a laugh.

The jam-packed lift comes to a juddering halt and the doors open to a sparse corridor leading to the ward. I've come to see a frail old lady requiring emergency abdominal surgery, and the heat of the ward hits me as I open the door to a bustling, busy atmosphere with lots of chatter and machines beeping. It's sort of exciting, popping back in. Moving to air-conditioned operating theatres was a dream, as was the change in work clothes. Anaesthetists work in scrubs, so now my entire work-life is destined to wake up in pyjamas, put on different pyjamas and work with people in primary-coloured pyjamas. Although the donning of uniform at hospital along with cycling enthusiasm has, I believe, fuelled the growing epidemic of middle-aged men in Lycra (MAMILs) in anaesthetics. I'm even starting to think Lycra is the grey hair of the underwear drawer, the shiny streaks building up the further you make it to retirement.

✛

After reading the notes and speaking to the nurse, I go to see Elsie, a pleasant elderly lady requiring surgery. She smiles and sits up as I arrive. There's a photo of her family on the table next to some well-wishing cards. Like most patients, she is visibly afraid of having an anaesthetic, so I sit with her and go through what will happen, reassuring where I can. When I ask about her teeth and if any are loose, she stares at her hands and then beckons me closer.

'Teeth?' she whispers, like we were doing a back-street deal.

'Yes,' I say. 'Any caps, crowns, bridges or dentures?'

She looks to check no one is about to come inside the curtain, then takes out her full dentures and pops them back in again.

'Please promise me one thing. If you take these out, please make sure I have my teeth back next to me after? My grandchildren, they don't know, they have never seen me without them. I don't want them to see it.'

It's at these moments in medicine where you're so preoccupied with making sure someone stays safe and alive, that something so human might not seem important, but let me tell you, it *really really* is.

It wasn't just the risks of an anaesthetic she was afraid of, but also the memories her family has of her, because when you lose control of everything, that includes the things we take for granted.

'Of course,' I reply. 'We'll make sure they're right beside you when you wake up.'

Every anaesthetic is uncharted territory for every patient. It's easy to forget that you juggle humanity with the adrenaline of the moment your anaesthetic takes their control away.

✚

As Christmas approaches, I decide to treat Dr Commons, by turning up looking swanky as. I proudly enter the hospital in full suit, waistcoat and tie that I recently wore to a friend's wedding. Slightly hot from all the commuting in this gear, I call out to him when I see him down the corridor. He turns, sees me approaching and for a second I see a smile come across his face. Is that a tear even?

'Well, well!' he says. 'Very impressive.'

As we both stand there in waistcoats, admiring our attire, a patient walks past, looking at us both.

'Bloody hell, it's Tweedledum and Tweedledee!'

Chapter 7

My first anaesthetics exam is coming up after about a year of anaesthetizing and I am truly learning the bizarre part of the science of this more occult syllabus. If you ever wondered whether medicine contains an element of dark magic to it, then let me tell you about the admittedly unmagical sounding heparin, which is a common blood-thinning agent used to treat or prevent blood clots. It's measured in 'international units', with one unit defined as the amount of heparin needed to keep a cat's blood wet for 24 hours at 0°C (32°F). And the antidote to heparin is protamine, made from none other than the sperm of fish. *How* do you collect fish sperm and *who* does that job? Maybe that's where the magic comes in? Would vegans object to having fish sperm save their life?

Alongside this, I am also discovering how to measure humidity using a strand of animal/human hair that then lengthens or shortens, or learning how erections are caused by the parasympathetic nervous system and ejaculation by the sympathetic nervous system (remembered as Point and Shoot, *very* important in anaesthetics).

I've reached a state of complete examination exhaustion and it's not as if failing prevents you from anaesthetizing the next day. You could fail, be in work after the results, possibly in a lower mood. You might start talking to your patient about feeling down and failing the exam, they might ask what the exam was for and just as you inject the sleepy anaesthetic drug:

'Well . . . for this really. Sweet dreams!'

This anaesthetics malarkey is not all just knocking people out in operating theatres. In fact, it is also our job to sometimes keep patients awake, on purpose. This is the case for Mildred, a frail old lady who has broken her ankle after slipping while gardening.

'Scared the life out of me, I tell you. I nearly kicked the dog on the way down.'

White hair and a warm smile, she's remarkably relaxed for the operation.

'Oh well, I've had a few operations in my time and survived. I assume you lot get better at what you're doing anyway.'

Due to her other health conditions, it has been deemed safer that we do the operation under a spinal anaesthetic, where we inject local anaesthetic and painkiller through a needle in the back, which makes her bottom half numb and also unable to move. This wears off, of course – it would be tricky discharging patients if it didn't.

Despite a spinal anaesthetic being considered safe and sometimes preferred to a general anaesthetic (GA), with benefits such as good pain relief, less risk to the lungs and less risk of confusion post-op, in the UK it's not uncommon to hear 'I don't want to be awake' responses from patients, with many requesting a GA irrespective as they would rather not be present (consciously at least) while we attempt to fix their body.

Mildred sits on the edge of the bed facing away from me since I need access to her back and spine. Scrubbed up, I give her skin a clean and apply a drape, feel for the top of her hips, then meet my thumbs across the middle to find a space between the spinal bones.

In patients with more insulation, it can be difficult to find these defined landmarks. One of my first times doing a spinal, I couldn't find the hip bones or spinal bones, no matter how hard I pushed. I turned to tell my consultant in a hushed voice so as not to offend by revealing the reason I cannot feel anything bony at all.

They looked at me matter-of-factly. 'Just have a go.'

Thankfully Mildred's bones are prominent, so I find a gap between a few moles with ease, in goes a little bit of local anaesthetic to numb the skin first, then I insert the long spinal needle through the skin, ligaments and soft tissue until the feeling of a slight 'pop', a tactile give on the needle. I look to see if I've got it in the right space and, sure enough, out comes some clear liquid that surrounds the brain, otherwise known as cerebrospinal fluid. In goes the anaesthetic and it's not long before she can't feel or move her legs and we're all set for some good old-fashioned bone carpentry.

A spinal does mean that you are required to up the small-talk game for a whole surgery as the patient is conscious and keen for some distracting natter. She begins with explaining how apologetic she is for wasting our time, but I assure her she most definitely isn't.

'My husband used to be an orthopaedic surgeon,' she says as the surgeons cut open her leg and get to work fixing her broken bones, while Mildred is completely unaware.

'Oh, didn't he offer to do your ankle?' I jest.

'No,' she laughed. 'He's dead.'

'Oh.'

'Lazy bugger he was anyway.'

Mildred chats away and I sit talking, occasionally marking down her vital signs. Eventually she asks if I'm married or have a partner.

'Well, you better get a move on,' she says firmly. I laugh and try to change the subject.

She persists in asking me more questions, so we go past the 'not met the right person' and 'still looking!' pleasantries to her digging deeper still. My consultant, Dr Shaif, pauses his crossword and tries to help out.

'The problem for Ed is there are just too many options.'

Options? Too many? What, like I'm some sort of Lothario wandering the hospital?

'It's true. If he doesn't get a move on, he'll be married to coffee and Lycra,' adds the orthopaedic surgeon as he hammers and drills into Mildred's leg.

What *is* this?

I hope the next patient has a general anaesthetic.

✚

Stepping out from the surgery, which became a cross-examination of my love life, or lack of, I hope my afternoon is less personal as I head into a pre-op clinic. It's here that patients who are high risk for operations are assessed to see how fit they are for surgery. It's one of the few times I have dressed up smart, knowing that I won't be in scrubs. Instead, I'm back in the Tweedledee outfit.

'Aha, my next subject,' Dr Cash exclaims as I enter the clinic room. I smile until I realize this isn't just his zany greeting.

'So, Ed. We've got a brand-new cardiopulmonary exercise machine.'

I look across to the exercise bike with all sorts of tech gizmos attached and pretend to look excited. Patients are asked to ride this, which then provides a detailed breakdown of their heart and lung physiology, helping inform fitness for surgery. It's quite an effort, so they are asked to come in loose/sporty clothing in preparation.

'We need some people to test it, so on you pop.'

'Me? I'm here for the clinic.'

'I know, lucky you are getting to try this too.'

Still unsure whether I want to do this, I'm guided onto the exercise bike by Dr Cash.

'I'm not exactly kitted up for exercise.'

'You'll be fine!' Dr Cash assures while hooking me up to his new machine.

Five minutes after entering this room, smartly dressed, I'm now drenched in sweat, tie on the floor, waistcoat hanging off the bicycle handle. Shirt open and untucked, with ECG leads dangling across my chest. A tight-fitting Darth-Vader-style mask drowns my lack-of-fitness pain in this gym-come-sauna.

'Come on, Ed! You've got *more*, I know it!'

After several minutes, which feel like hours, I beg for mercy and slump in the chair, breathless, having nearly passed out on the machine, sweat still pouring, after I've kicked my shoes off in order to prevent blisters from forming. A nurse arrives at the door with a patient.

'Oh, sorry, I didn't realize you still had a patient with you, Dr Cash.'

'No, no, don't worry, that's just Ed, one of the trainees,' he says. 'Come on in and have a seat, Ed needs a few minutes to recover in the corner there.'

✚

Anaesthetic presence is pretty much ubiquitous across hospital, working with patients of every age: in clinics for pain or pre-op; in Psychiatry, giving patients anaesthetic for electroconvulsive therapy; or at emergencies such as cardiac arrests and collapsed patients; or if the hospital runs out of coffee.

Another area leads me to follow in old John Snow's footsteps once again. As a side project to his cholera heroics, John went on to become a pioneer in the little-known discipline of anaesthesia, famously administering chloroform to Queen Victoria to assist the delivery of Prince Leopold. It was so successful that the concept of childbirth anaesthesia was also born. Given the royal approval, Snow was invited back for a second gig and helped the Queen to deliver Princess Beatrice.

Fittingly for my John Snow tribute act, I, too, am delivering anaesthetic to a Beatrice (not royal but probably related), who has booked the delivery of one's baby via Caesarean section.

'Ohhhhhhhhhhh, you must be our anaesthetist,' Beatrice giggles and surprises all of us with an accidental snort. She and her husband are both terribly excited and talk to me like I am a wine sommelier with exclusive vintages on offer. I take the role of drug sommelier and go through orders of the day.

'To summarize: cannula in the hand, a spinal anaesthetic, followed by the delivery of one baby, how does that sound?'

Beatrice laughs with full home-county guffaw and clasps her hands excitedly around her mouth. I turn, holding my hand out like a waiter to the husband.

'And for you, sir?'

They both laugh.

I hate myself.

A planned Caesarean section is probably the most joyous anaesthetic we can give, as at the end of it there's a baby. When it's an emergency C-section, it can be much more stressful. It wasn't planned and now the surgeons need the baby out within 30 minutes. So, pleasantries go out the window as you introduce yourself in the corridor while the mum is wheeled down to theatre, to talk about putting a needle in her back or having to go to sleep because there isn't time for a spinal anaesthetic. If things go well, it's incredible, but it can be devastatingly heart-breaking when it doesn't.

During my first C-section, cognitively exhausted by learning the anaesthetic technique, I am running on endorphins when the midwife brings over a newborn baby to the tearful, happy couple. It's a special moment.

'Would you mind, a photo?' They hand me their phone.

'It would be my pleasure!' I beam, then get in position and snap.

It's only when I see their expressions that I realize they meant a photo of just the three of them, *not* a selfie with me.

＋

Spinals and epidurals are the general orders of the day from anaesthetists working in obstetrics, the latter being a similar needle-in-the-back experience but not pushed as far (into the epidural space) and a small catheter threaded through, which can provide ongoing pain relief for mum while she is in labour. That's why I'm called to one of the delivery rooms and also where I meet Josie, a midwife, for the first time. Josie opens the door and I suddenly find my speaking is jumbled.

'Hi, I . . . '

'Epidural?' she says.

'Yes, that's me.'

Something in my stomach is churning, but I try to ignore it and not look at Josie again. I'm *not* a teenager. I get everything ready and position the pregnant lady, Rebecca, with help from her husband.

'Just relax for me,' I say to Rebecca, currently in labour and therefore totally incapable of doing anything remotely like relaxing. She lets out an ear-piercing scream with the next contraction and Josie raises her eyebrows at me.

'Once we get the epidural in, we'll be able to relax.'

The top of the hips are again not easy to find. Trying my best to concentrate, I go through the routine and manage to get the needle into the right place and thread the catheter. Delighted that I've not messed this up, I turn to see if Josie is equally impressed, essentially at me just doing my job, but she's not watching me, she is watching Rebecca's husband, who collapses to the floor fainting with a thud. Great, more work.

I pop back a while later to check if the epidural is working and find Rebecca comfortable and smiling, while her husband has some colour back in his cheeks.

✚

Josie and I work a few more shifts together and my nervousness in her presence does not ease.

In fact, it appears to increase. A few weeks later, we're walking out of hospital together and I find myself saying something unexpected.

'I was wondering if . . . you would like to . . . '

At the last minute I bail out.

'. . . fill out a feedback form for me? It only takes a minute. Just got to get a few bits of feedback from all over, you know!'

Really, Ed? What a catch you are, giving out the joy of admin to people.

'Of course, here's my email.'

She writes it down on a scrap and hands it to me.

'Great and . . . '

I nearly bail again, but with no get-out this time and the memory of Mildred and the merry band of bone carpenters grilling me, I persevere against better judgement.

'and . . . and I just wondered, if you'd be interested, I mean no worries if not, in, errr . . . '

'Going for a drink?' she guesses.

'Yes . . . yes, exactly that,' I say.

'I'd love to.'

'What? WOW . . . I mean . . . great! So . . . '

'Well, you've got my email now.'

'Yes, I'll email you for . . . email for a DATE.' I cringe at myself. *Stop* talking, Ed.

'I look forward to it,' she smiles and turns towards her car.

'Check your junk mail,' I say as she walks away.

My mind was screaming.

ED, YOU FOOL. STOP IT. NOW.

✚

I'm soon starting a run of night shifts and, truth be told, I like them. It's where you really find independence, with the on-call consultant at home unless you need to bother them. The hospital becomes a different, enchanting place too. The hubbub of daily life dies down and the skeleton staff of night shift means the corridors feel so much longer and wider. As I walk down the main corridor, I spot a porter who whistles '*Nessun dorma*' at the other end, rising to such a dramatic, echoey climax as I pass that I join in and we continue to duet as I head towards theatres.

I've also started to develop my own personal quirks and preferences, too. Drawing up my drugs and positioning them in a blue tray, horizontal for the initial anaesthetic drugs, straight on for other medicine like anti-sickness and painkillers. I fill a red tray with all the emergency drugs, just in case the blood pressure is too low, if the heart beats too slowly, plus also adrenaline in case of cardiac arrest or anaphylaxis. *Plan for the worst, hope for the best* is the mantra of anaesthetics.

Early on in my career, I'd be slightly terrified of injecting powerful anaesthetic drugs into patients, with a general fear that anything you touch might lead to you accidentally killing someone. Now there's the reassurance that it won't – well, not immediately. Now it feels as comfortable as making toast.

Because our drugs go into veins, anaesthetists need intravenous access almost all the time, so we're generally the go-to people if the nurses and doctors on the ward struggle to get cannulas into patients with difficult veins (with a general rule that you ask your own senior first before calling anaesthetics). Either way, just being polite generally gets you places. Not what I get when bleeped by a new FY1 doctor on the ward.

'Hi, anaesthetist.'

Hi, anaesthetist?

'I can't get a cannula in and my senior is busy, they're in an operation, so you need to come now?' came a rude tone.

'OK, and who are you?'

'I'm the new junior doctor on the surgical ward. Could you come now so we can give the antibiotics? My senior is busy, in the middle of an operation.'

'You said. Well, I could, but I think your senior would be *very* angry.'

'And *why* is that exactly?' came the impatient reply.

'Well, his patient will wake up.'

'What are you talki . . . ohh, umm.' The phone hangs up.

✚

At least being called 'anaesthetist' was a break from my near-daily explanation of my name to people on the phone.

'Patrick. Yes, that is my second name. Yes . . . yes, I know it's also a first name. It's Ed Pat . . . Ed is my . . . Yes. No no, not Patrick Ed, it's Ed Patrick.'

'Ah, got you!' comes the voice over the phone. 'Thanks, Patrick.'

Chapter 7

✚

Deep into the night shift, an appendix needs to come out, so I go to see Sanjay, a man in his 30s, stocky, muscular, crew-cut hair and owner of said appendix. Despite also being the owner of several tattoos, he reports feeling uneasy around needles, surprisingly not an uncommon phenomenon among tattoo bearers. While everyone around him sleeps, we go through the pre-op routine, but through whispered voices so we don't wake up everyone around us, not that anyone can sleep deeply in hospital.

Austin the ODP and I get everything ready and soon Sanjay is brought into the anaesthetic room. I try my best to relax people before an anaesthetic, so we get chatting and I see him calm, the monitor shows his heart rate becomes a little slower and Sanjay asks if someone can play a song off his phone when he wakes up, 'Heaven is a Halfpipe'.

'Sure.'

I ask what he does for a living to continue the relaxed vibe.

'I'm a plasterer.'

'Ooh, I've been looking for a plasterer for ages!' I say excitedly as I inject anaesthetic.

'Well, now seems like a pretty good time to negotiate a price,' pipes Austin, followed by a spike in Sanjay's blood pressure.

'At least you won't need those emergency drugs, Ed.'

Once he's anaesthetized, I look with the laryngoscope for the dark hole and Sanjay's vocal cords but I can only see a small part of them. I ask Austin for a bougie (a sort of stretched-out plastic coat hanger that works as a guidewire). In it goes, and we railroad the breathing tube into the right place, then take the coat hanger out. I flick the ventilator switch and turn on anaesthetic gases, then place a tie round the back of Sanjay's head to fix the tube in place with as it pokes out of his mouth. Austin tapes Sanjay's eyes shut, protecting them from sterile drapes and anything that might brush across his face.

The surgeons waltz in and I spend the next hour filling out notes, tweaking gas levels and giving more medicines, and being forced to listen to a general surgeon's playlist.

When the operation comes to an end, I grab the suction tubing and suck out any drool or secretions from Sanjay's mouth and we wait for him to wake up, the beeping monitor now the only noise. Austin hits 'play' on Sanjay's phone just as he is waking up. 'Heaven is a Halfpipe' starts playing.

'If I die before I wake . . . '

'Actually, Austin, skip that one.'

After Sanjay has woken and gone back to the ward, I start to doze off on the staffroom couch. My bleep goes off, putting an end to dreams of sleeping.

Adult cardiac arrest, A&E resus. ETA 10 minutes

As the on-call anaesthetist with skills in managing airways and cardiovascular support, you are needed at almost any emergency, especially in those instances where your skills are needed for someone not breathing. I make my way to resus, where all the sickest people in hospital arrive, and get ready at the head end of the bed with the breathing equipment. I am waiting along with a team of nurses and doctors.

Details phoned in to the A&E red phone by the ambulance crew were scarce: a young adult male found in water.

We stand and wait, a hushed silence comes over us before the patient arrives through the double doors, pushed in on a trolley as a paramedic continues CPR onto the lifeless body. I'm taken aback as the man is young, younger than a lot of patients I've anaesthetized, maybe younger than Sanjay. We transfer him quickly to the hospital bed, and that's when I start to realize, he's dead. The skin is ice cold. Oxygen is attached, I suction the airway for fluid and I start hand ventilating.

CPR continues in a futile effort to pump blood around the heart. Another doctor tries to get blood from what looks like an engorged vein, but nothing comes as the blood is solid, congealed. The moment to save this life passed a long time ago and we are all just realizing this. Nothing on the monitors and no clinical signs of life. After a while, the consultant who is leading calls an end to our efforts and I squeeze the last ever breath to enter these lungs. We turn the body to check for any signs of injury, and more water pours out the mouth.

Fuck.

You expect the unexpected in medicine, but that doesn't mean you're immune from the effects.

I've seen countless unconscious patients, but driving home after that shift, I realize it's the faces of people that don't wake up that will stay with me forever.

Chapter 8

Wake me up
before you go-go . . .

The surgeon has left his playlist running and George Michael is now blaring. In retrospect, I should have turned the anaesthetic gas off sooner, as now everyone is waiting. The scrub team needing to clean the theatre are waiting, the surgeons are bumming around waiting, the next patient on the ward is waiting, all while Taylor and I wait for Mo, our current patient, to wake up. Waiting for him to blow off enough sevoflurane (anaesthetic gas) that he notices the rather large breathing tube sat in his throat and feels compelled to take it out. It's better this way round, after the operation has finished. No one wants to wake up before then. Still, no one wants to hang around while the slow-coach anaesthetist here takes an age to wake up his patients. It's a balance.

My drugs tray sits on the machine next to me, full of discarded empty syringes, the patient notes next to that. The operating theatre is otherwise deserted. Taylor and I have exhausted our chat for now, so we both enjoy the quiet, aside from the music.

Waiting.

Not that dilly-dallying is new to me. My overanalytical and overthinking mind has been hard at work for many years, taking extra time to decide anything from buying new mugs in IKEA (two hours I spent wondering what rim is best, followed only then by the handle and radius dimensions), to making life decisions, like medicine.

I also took too much time (stretching to several hours) trying to construct the perfect message, or email, to Josie.

Our first date is at the cinema, a classic, non-speaking date. I buy a massive tub of popcorn after being indecisive about the sizes and deciding to essentially have all of them in one. But I make the most of it during the movie, while also checking Josie isn't watching me ungainly shovelling popcorn into my mouth and spilling it all over my lap and the floor.

Afterwards, I drop her off and as we're talking in the car, there's that tangible moment where we're slightly invading each other's personal space. Is there a, dare I say it, *kiss* about to happen? We both lean towards each other, and just as something is about to happen:

'UGHHHUURRRRGGGHHHH!' The sound comes unexpectedly from my mouth, as Josie looks on, worried.

'Are you OK?'

'I've got cramp . . . in my leg, hang on . . . '

'I thought you were having a seizure!'

I open the door and stumble out, then push against the car to stretch out my leg and the cramp.

'Ahhh, phew.'

Josie gets out the car.

'Are you OK? It's getting a bit late, I best go and get ready for work tomorrow.'

Damn those lack of electrolytes that have just ruined my date.

'Let's do it again, though, I had a great time,' she adds.

'Yes!' I say, with such springing vigour the cramp resumes.

✚

I look at the anaesthetic machine beeping away. The oxygen levels sit at 100 per cent, the heart rate and blood pressure are unconcerning, and importantly the level of anaesthetic gas in Mo's lungs is finally getting low enough for him to wake up. Seconds after this thought crosses my mind, Mo suddenly sits bolt upright, with a startle in his eyes.

'OK, Mo, OK, let's take this out then.'

I take the breathing tube out as he stares at me. He takes a couple of breaths.

'Bloody hell, that's a bit big,' Mo croaks, before he puts his head back on the pillow and starts snoozing.

I finish up and take Mo round to the recovery, where patients are monitored further and, when recovered more, sent back to the ward. Quickly I grab some food from the canteen and eat it on my way, walking across the hospital to some other operating theatres where my rota has me down for a children's dental list this afternoon. With my experience in paediatrics, I'm aware of how the rapport building and deal brokering goes in order to do what you need.

'I just need to have a look in your ears and mouth.'

'No.'

'You'll get a sticker for being brave?'

'Mmm. OK, deal.'

The difference with children in anaesthetics is that the stakes are higher for me. Having that rapport and doing the anaesthetic as gently and smoothly as possible is the aim. Easy does it. In an ideal world, small children would always be amenable to having an anaesthetic and drift off to sleep like adults, no fuss. It does happen, but the cannulas, masks, strange-smelling anaesthetic gases and these weird-looking anaesthetic people mean the opposite happens too. So there can be tears, upset and kicking the anaesthetist where it hurts. So we try to gain rapport at every moment, gain that trust. Tommy is first on the dental list, six years old.

'I don't like needles.'

'Me neither!' I say, trying to show we're buddies, on the same team.

'He won't let a needle near him without screaming the place down,' his mum explains.

We agree to a deal of gas induction, where instead of having a cannula and drugs injected, Tommy will breathe through a funny-smelling mask while sitting with Mummy, and hopefully he'll anaesthetize himself in doing so, and not Mum.

✚

I prepare drugs in the anaesthetic room, in smaller syringes as smaller doses are needed. Dr Cash, fresh from giving my body a flogging on the exercise bike, has another challenge for me.

'Ed, here.' He chucks me a glove.

'Make a unicorn.'

'A what?' I say, stretching out the glove.

'I'm off to get Tommy. Blow that up and draw a unicorn. It'll be fun for him, keep him distracted.'

With the unexpected task, I take the blue glove and blow into the end, until it inflates to a decent but not about-to-pop size. How do I draw a unicorn? I also realize I can't draw. But without any other options, I take the permanent marker and haphazardly draw some eyes around one of the fingers, eyebrows, a mouth with teeth, ears and a nose. It looks a bit odd to me and just as I'm wondering what to do with it, Dr Cash comes in with Tommy and his mum.

'And look what Dr Ed has made you! He's made you a unico . . . '

Dr Cash sees me holding my unicorn attempt and smiling, but his expression goes from feigning excitement to horror. He grabs my unicorn and surreptitiously throws it in the bin.

'Bloody hell, Ed, we don't want to give him nightmares,' he whispers.

'I tried!'

All of us are super-excited and making the atmosphere as fun as possible, with that fake, overt enthusiasm adults tend to perform in front of children. Because we all want it to be calm, the atmosphere is a bit tense, like being around a mafia boss, trying not to make them angry so they don't dispose of you. Tommy, the mafia boss, looks at me unmoved. He is already considering whether to have me whacked.

Tommy is going along with everything, slightly suspicious, rightly so. He's got his henchman, Berty the bunny, right by his side. No one messes with them.

To make things as easy as possible, Tommy sits on his mum's knee with a tablet, watching cartoons. His mum makes murmurings of everything being perfectly fine and normal, just a day out, and that these nice people are going to sort his teeth. But Tommy and Berty look around, not so sure. After getting everything ready, Dr Cash gives me a nod to bring in the mask and turn on some gases from the anaesthetic machine. Placing it slowly below Tommy's chin while he watches the screen, the hope is he'll breathe in enough to start falling unconscious. After a few seconds, he looks down and sees the mask, then up at me. A few tense seconds, but he goes back to the cartoons.

'You're doing really well, Tommy. Just holding this mask here. You carry on watching, with Berty.'

He looks around and holds Berty tight. The bunny's arm pops out towards me like he's fending me off.

Slowly, Tommy becomes drowsy in mum's arms, and wriggles a

little. I place one hand to support the back of his head and use my other to lift his chin into the mask. His eyes start to roll, the room fills with the smell of anaesthetic gases that are leaking around the mask. Eventually he goes floppy, Dr Cash steps in and, with the help of mum and me, we move Tommy onto the bed.

Tears roll down his cheek, but they're not from Tommy. His mum is in tears. Mum strokes Tommy's hairline and kisses his forehead, as I use the mask and bag to squeeze some breaths for him. She says goodbye and thanks us all, leaving with the support of the nurse to get a much-needed cup of tea. Almost every parent cries at this moment, I haven't seen one that hasn't yet. You have to ask your child to trust you and then watch as they stop breathing.

'You call *that*' – Dr Cash points to the bin – ' . . . a *unicorn*?'

'I, well, I'm not the most artistic admittedly.'

'You scared me, let alone a six-year-old. Right, let's take him through to theatre.'

✚

Once we're all set up in the operating theatre, I sit, looking forward to some downtime making notes, planning my next text to Josie.

'No, no, Ed. You've still got to hold the head,' Dr Cash breaks my daydream.

'Hold the head?'

'Yes, for the dentist, for traction.'

I move my chair and sit right next to Tommy's head in front of the anaesthetic machine that his breathing is hooked up to. I hold his head steady from the sides as the dentist starts to pull teeth out. It's an awkward position and my back starts to ache, more work than I initially thought. Then come the sounds. The sound of hearing a child's teeth crack and grind is enough to make you a bit queasy. Add that I can feel the vibrations through Tommy's skull of teeth being extracted, well, this is certainly one of my least favourite things. Teeth and blood are removed from Tommy's mouth as the dentist works away. I grimace and look to the side, where Berty the bunny is sat glaring at me.

✚

As I'm waiting for the last patient to wake up, my arms aching from holding heads while teeth are taken out, the crash bleep goes off.

Adult cardiac arrest. Ward 24

I'm keeping a cardiac-arrest team waiting because I can't leave an anaesthetized patient, so I wait until they're awake before quickly joining the rest of the arrest team on the ward. A hub of people hold crash bleeps (that alert the holder to hospital emergencies), such as medical teams, resus teams, anaesthetists and intensive-care doctors, so someone should be there. I waddle fast through the hospital, hot from the unexpected exercise, and by the time I arrive, I've got a stitch. There is a full resus going on. The ICU doctors have intubated, someone is doing chest compressions, another doctor tries to get more IV access. The three other curtains in the bay are closed to patients, who must rightly be terrified. I go round to the head end and take over the breathing duties. The patient, Doris, is 78 years old. Chest compressions continue, adrenaline goes in, no signs of life on the monitor, no pulse, nothing. We carry on for a while longer, different people switch in to do chest compressions, but nothing changes. The ICU doctor leading the resus calls an end and asks if anyone objects. No one objects, we stop and I stop making breaths for her. She's still. People file out from the bed space and nurses come to look after Doris one final time. As I walk out, I hear one of the ward doctors.

'It's so sad, her husband died not long ago, they were married for over 50 years.'

Leaving the ward, I wonder if there might have been a broken-heart syndrome going on (known as Takotsubo cardiomyopathy). It causes the heart to become enlarged and weakened, and can be brought on by extremely stressful events, like bereavement. You *really* can have a broken heart.

Fifty years. Fifty years with the same person, the same soul. It's all you'd ever know. And then, gone, alone. Fifty years, I can't imagine it, it would take me fifty years to decide on fifty years. How do those relationships start?

✚

On call that evening and soon to finish, I receive a bleep from the urology surgeon.

'I've got a fractured penis.'

'So sorry to hear that.'

He ignores me while my brain remembers that this organ does not contain any bones. It's an injury that occurs during blunt trauma, usually through overenthusiastic sex. Imagine thrusting against a brick wall.

'We need to operate later tonight.'

'Oh, well, um.'

'Is something wrong?'

'Well, I've been told it has to be life- or limb-saving surgery for overnight operations. Hang on, let me check.'

I wander around the theatre complex, looking for Dr Cash, but also asking various people a philosophical question: what counts as a limb?

'Yep, no problem. Apparently, a penis *does* count as a limb.'

Chapter 9

'Now put the speculum in the eye.'

I look around, confused. Luckily for George, our awake patient, the consultant, Sally, means a small wire retractor to keep the eyelids open, not a vaginal speculum.

I place it under George's top and bottom eyelid, the speculum then holds them back, exposing his eyeball, and prevents him from blinking.

'Now in the corner towards the nose, grab a piece of his eye with the forceps, *good*.

'Cut that layer of the eye open, *good*.

'Now use the blunt forceps to go into it, *yep, good*.

'Now push them back around the eyeball, a bit further, *that's it*.'

Even I winced. There was a slight squelching sound too. *Push them back around the eyeball?!*

There's something unsettling about anaesthetizing eyes, the way they just, well, *look* at you.

'Are you OK, George?' I say, feeling queasy myself.

'Good, thanks, as long as you're not taking out my eye.'

'Not yet . . . ' Sally interjects. 'Now, Ed, needle in behind the eyeball, *good*.

'And inject anaesthetic, *good!*

'*Now* your eye is ready for taking out, George. Well, the cataract is. All done, sorry for talking all that through, it was Ed's first time doing that block.'

'Just as well I couldn't see then.'

We push George on the trolley into theatre for the final case of the day. As the ophthalmologist finishes, everyone starts cleaning and departs, but I hang around to finish my online statutory mandatory training on a computer, the bane of health-care workers.

'Not leaving?' Sally says, grabbing her bag and coat from underneath the sink, a favourite storage space in the anaesthetic room.

'Stat man,' I frown.

'Ohhh, well, don't go home too late now,' Sally waves and I'm left with the NHS computer still logging in.

Stat man, a boxset series of mind-numbingly dull modules of videos and questions everyone has to complete. At my old NHS trust I kept failing a part because I didn't know the different temperatures that mop heads need to be washed at. I must have missed that class at medical school. I click through to the module on Fire Safety and see the first question.

What is fire?

Seriously.

Why is this even a question?

I'll go out on a limb and say that if a doctor didn't know what fire was, then they shouldn't be a doctor. Even cavemen would reject them. I roll my eyes and pull out my phone for some procrastination.

✚

I took my anaesthetics exam recently, opting to take it in Birmingham, where curiously it was held at the Birmingham Botanical Gardens.

I get there early to walk around the gardens and calm my nerves. Everywhere there are peacocks. Two are atop of the gates. They are inside too, hiding among plants and anaesthetists revising last minute. When I am called into the hall, I have to skip past three peacocks just to get in.

'Could you shut the door behind you? We don't want the peacocks coming in,' the exam invigilator asks, shaking a roll of paper at a nonplussed peacock.

I never imagined that peacocks could be a hazard for an exam. Maybe I'd get a free resit if I failed, though? Because failing is expensive. Doctors in every specialty have to pay for their exams, £350 for this one alone. If you fail, you have to pay again, and again and again. The bills can mount up.

The hall is dark. Adorned with left-over decorations from weddings and other celebrations, it doesn't really have an exam atmosphere, more a morning-after-the-disco vibe. I sit down and start the three-hour exam, immediately making a fist bump as I see a question on fish sperm come up.

A few weeks later, I log on to the results page, a simple list of candidate numbers with only the words PASS highlighted in blue or FAIL highlighted in red, I nervously scroll down and among a block of red, a single blue pass box sits next to my number.

Yes!

Passed!

My prize for passing, you ask? Well, getting ready for *more* exams.

Chapter 9

Things are going well with Josie, too. I've progressed from formal emailing to informal texting. She has also given me excellent work feedback, so in retrospect that admin request was a good move even if it hadn't worked out.

'Some excellent comments here, Ed,' says my supervisor, signing off my annual feedback. 'You really have impressed someone!'

Cinema and Nando's goes a long way.

I've also won approval from one of Josie's important family members. Not her parents, but Nelly, a chocolate cockapoo. Having always wanted a dog, I am determined to impress. Admittedly Nelly's approval is won with almost anything edible, but not having it would amount to end of romance, so this is as vital as passing the anaesthetics exam.

Josie has moved to a different hospital, too, so we only see each other outside of our antisocial shifts, meaning a lot of our messages are the 'How's your day?' or 'What are you eating? Can I have some?' type of messages.

Today I receive:

'Are you worried about this?'

She's sent along a link to a news article. I've seen a few similar news pieces and other online chatter too.

I look back at the computer screen.

What is fire?

I wonder this philosophically: what *is* fire? Destruction? Rage? An order?

I hit 'reveal answer'. Ooh the excitement.

Fire is the visible effect of smoke, heat and flames

No shit, well, I guess I'll see it coming.

I go back to the news article. The truth is I'm not worried about it, plus the last time I thought an infectious disease was going to cause havoc I ended up buying a lifetime's supply of tuna and pasta. I'm not making that mistake again.

An email from Dr Cash pops up on the screen. Wow, I *am* popular this evening.

Emergency meeting tomorrow for all trainee anaesthetists after teaching

Maybe I will pick up some pasta on the way home.

✚

I, like everyone else, had no knowledge or concern about a deadly virus when it arrived in Europe. However, samples from sewers in Italy on 18 December 2019 showed the virus was already brewing there. Just in time for their Christmas dinner. In the UK we were tucking into an election turkey complete with a good stuffing and were all completely oblivious to the threat. Just how every good horror movie foretells.

✚

As I take a seat, an uncomfortable one at that, in the anaesthetics office after our weekly teaching session, I realize I am slightly sweaty, due to my only-quality-caffeine-will-do addiction and rushing off to a nearby barista. Dr Cash leads what, I realize in retrospect, is the battle talk as I flip open my flat white, replete with a heart pattern on the foam.

'You've all probably heard about Covid-19.'

There is a palpable excitement. Until now, it was simply rumouring from Italy, internet stories, Twitter and other social-media posts. All of it hyped up and ridiculous. Finally, we are going to hear the truth and reality from our senior sources. So when the exact same internet and Twitter posts pop up in the presentation,

I am gobsmacked. Because everything I've read *is* true. The average citizen knows just as much as me, *a doctor*. There was no hyperbole, it is real. The only new information we have is the timeframe to it hitting the UK hard.

'Two weeks.

'Then we need all airway-trained doctors who are young, and therefore supposedly lower risk, in intensive care. That's you lot. I realize this sounds scary. It's uncharted territory for all of us, no one has faced anything like this before, but we'll try to support you as much as possible.'

✚

We don't have to wait long for trepidation. Dr Cash goes through the dos and don'ts for intubating Covid-19 patients.

In short, every anaesthetist knows the Difficult Airway (DAS) guidelines for when you run into trouble putting a breathing tube in. A series of steps you take, working down an algorithm, helping you focus to prevent someone dying in front of you.

The very, very, *very* last step is to cut open the neck and put a breathing tube in that way.

It's messy, plus shit has properly hit the fan if this is happening. Speak to the most experienced anaesthetists and only a few will have ever done or seen this. I once had a go on a pig's neck – a dead one, so I can't even tell you if they lived.

Dr Cash gestures to the new guidelines on screen.

'You use a video laryngoscope, you have one attempt, then cut open the neck.'

What?

One attempt, then straight to slicing a neck open?

'The information we have is that we don't have time, these patients desaturate and die quickly. The other thing to mention is to look after yourselves, no heroics. No PPE, don't go in. If someone says, for example, "Doctor, it's a 34-year-old woman with three kids and she's gonna die unless you intubate", no, you do NOT go in.

'**Understood?**

'There are only so many of you and if you lot go down, we'll lose this pretty quickly.'

I've never heard anything like it, my mouth hangs open as a single word repeatedly runs through my head.

'Fuck, Fuck, Fuck, Fuck, Fuck, Fuck, Fuck Fuck Fuck Fuck.'

Then, out of nowhere, he puts a pig's neck on the table.

'Right, who wants to have a go?'

Even David Cameron would have flinched.

Chapter 10

Big changes were about to happen in my life.

One of them is the pandemic about to hit our shores.

And the other is that Josie is moving in with me after our relationship was deemed a success.

✚

Moving in along with Josie are of course Nelly, plus two Maine Coon cats, Stormy and Peanut, which means getting used to some new routines. Animals seem to need feeding every morning, indeed they *expect* it. Catering duties lie with the person getting up for work first.

So, as I roll downstairs one early spring morning, I realize that person is me. What I don't allow time for is getting animals *inside* for breakfast, a rookie mistake. Peanut, to his credit, is already here, because food is all he desires. Stormy, however, is nowhere to be seen and Nelly is still outside after her morning relief, hurtling around the garden. It's taking longer than usual to get Nelly in, so I step outside, topless, into the cold morning as it starts raining, with pimples raising across my torso to a crescendo of my nipples saluting the misty air.

At 6am it feels strangely liberating, explaining loudly into the garden why I need to get into hospital quickly. Nelly considers my monologue, takes a breath, which adds to the mist, and turns to bark at a tree. After a few minutes she suddenly sprints towards the doorway. My pleading face turns to relief as finally I have coaxed her in. Then, at the last moment, she veers away back into the garden, clearly the dog version of pretending to throw a ball but not releasing it. Peanut meanwhile has started to help himself to *my* breakfast.

'Oi! You little shit,' I usher him off the counter.

Nelly finally comes in and I shut the door. Then I remember Stormy isn't inside, so back outside I go, where the heavens have opened. For a few minutes I shake some cat biscuits while shouting 'Stormy, Stormy!', still topless. Before one of my perplexed neighbours opens their window and shouts.

'Can you shut the fuck up, Rainman? It's 6AM.'

After the drive to hospital, I'm still late and such is my rush, I haven't found time to tie my shoes. Since I'm changing into crocs in 60 yards, I waddle into hospital like a child not ready for school, bypassing the newly free bacon sandwiches and down the corridor to the run-down changing room. This tiny room is suitable for about eight people but serves around eighty of us. There is also a shower attached to the room, which is poorly ventilated, so steam fills the place whenever anyone is showering and it starts to feel like an illegal staff sauna. I don't need to spell it out, but you can forget social distancing here.

After managing to get scrubs on while elbowing three other staff members as I pull on my trousers, I scurry to handover in the large lecture theatre. We've moved handover here as it's the only place where some sort of distancing can work (assuming none of us caught Covid-19 while changing).

On the way to the auditorium, I pass an old advert for paintball. I remember being forced to play it at a friend's stag do, as if *attending* a stag do wasn't punishment enough. The process involves donning cumbersome protective equipment, having safety rules shouted at you and being randomly assigned to a team. 'Team' is a strong word, because we were put into the battlefield for some *Fortnite*-style carnage. No one cared what or who they hit, everyone had spent a fortune on pricey paintballs and was determined to get their money's worth. I felt sorry for the trees, splattered in paint while hungover revellers pelted anything to unload their ammunition. The rule was to put your hand up once hit, which was a relief because I could sit out the rest. I realize Covid-19 is the new paintball, with that same constant lingering hangover feeling, cumbersome equipment and no one wanting to get hit.

✚

Everything in hospital soon becomes a military operation, thanks largely to Dr Carl Jenkinson, one of the anaesthetic registrars. He also works for the army and has just arrived back from an expedition in South America. Back in Blighty, he is leading a task force for the ICU set-up in the hospital and has already started a battle-style presentation. As I enter, Carl pauses while I, the hapless Private Patrick, find a seat.

'Sorry, animal issues,' I whisper.

Carl continues, occasionally pointing things out with a personalized wooden stick pointer he always carries, more for status than necessity.

'Obveeeeeously our enemy heeeerre is Covid-19, and preparation eeees key. What the enemeeey does not know helps us.'

He flings the wooden stick about as slides roll, the inflections in his voice surprising everyone as they hit extremes. You're unlikely to fall asleep for long during his talks.

When he moves on to ICU expansion in the hospital, everyone sits up. He's made a graphic of the current ICU floor plan and a new temporary one, located on a ward we are stealing from the medical team. Overall, it means the capacity of ICU beds increasing from twelve to around forty. For each thirteen-hour shift (day or night) there will be four anaesthetists or airway doctors, which Carl represents by four moving dots in each unit. We'll be put into teams and work the same pattern.

'Two of you will be positioned heehar, the other two heehar,' he flicks the wooden stick across.

'Should our defences be breached and we lose an airway doctor . . . '

He removes one of the red dots, which is ominously replaced by a skull and crossbones.

' . . . we will only have two or three on a sheeeft, so split yourselves according to cleenical situation.' The remaining red dots start moving frantically.

✚

He reaches the end and reads out the teams we'll be in. Which team have we got?

'Red team: Grabban, Patrick, Worrall.'

Ah, fuck, you're kidding?

Worrall. One of those slightly annoying, passive-aggressive personalities with a tendency to make you feel small. During a recent training session we were asked a specific question on intubating pregnant women. Worrall loudly scoffed during my answer to the consultant, then reeled off his opposing view, only for me to be proven right and him wrong. He didn't apologize, instead just stared thin-lipped at my colourful crocs, which I twirled to showcase my deep enjoyment.

He doesn't like coffee either, so why he chose anaesthetics I've no idea.

✚

Louisa Grabban, however, is all-round great and the most senior out of us three. An experienced registrar, she had taken time out of training, avoiding the rat race to becoming a consultant for a better work–life balance, something hard to come by in medicine. She's been at this hospital for a long time and seen many anaesthetists come and go, which means she is privy to *all* the gossip. During a night shift together, she gleefully filled me in on the history of my on-call room that night.

'Oh, you're in RB42?! That room has seen a *lot*!' before telling me the story of a plastic surgeon and an anaesthetist that decided to work on some anatomy behind closed doors. It always amazes me that despite hospital being such a dirty and manky place, lusty tendencies still endure. It's not getting an STI I'd be worried about, it's a splinter.

✚

But hang on, that's only three of us? Before I realize it, I'm saying my thought out loud.

'That's only three?'

Carl approaches me like the new recruit who needs to drop and give him 20.

'Yeeeees, uneven numbers, Ed, so the maths doesn't fit. Not ideal, but hopefully some locum cover will plug theeee gaps.'

Carl quickly moves on to how we are 'strengthening our defences'. Other doctors and nurses will be redeployed to ICU, food will be provided on site and car-parking charges scrapped.

We will be using radios to communicate between the 'dirty'

and 'clean' zones, leading several teams to start bidding for *Top Gun*-inspired radio aliases.

'Look, we can't all be Dr Goose or Maverick,' I hear one of my colleagues say.

✚

I become acutely aware of every surface people touch in hospital. With the virus rumoured to survive for a lengthy time on any surface, we could never be sure what surface was clean and whether we were still carrying the virus on our person. People lean on door frames or walls, type on multi-user computers, sit on chairs and touch the handles, rifle through patient notes and use the microwave. I had already decided to give up on finger food in hospital, meaning no more crisps or sandwiches. The ICU doctors' office lies several doors away from the nearest sink, which means washing my hands, then guarding them through several sets of doors, before finally opening some Pringles once inside the office and shovelling them into my mouth. It feels too much, doing a sterile procedure for such a short-lived potato snack.

At home, there is also a new routine to get to grips with, our new 'porch system'. It is the one place Josie and I implement a Covid-19 house change, creating a low-key air lock. Everything outside is treated as a risk if returning from hospital, because we can never be sure we aren't covered in coronavirus. Even after washing your hands in hospital, you again have to go through several sets of doors, touching handles all the way, meaning you question both your hands' cleanliness and whether a hospital needs this many doors.

✚

So, in order to keep our home Covid 'clean', the air lock serves as a place for us to strip off completely, while the other person holds back excited animals so we can go straight into the shower.

Upon returning home from work in the evening, I begin to ungainly strip to rid myself of any contamination I may have picked up from work. Josie has forgotten to unlock the inner porch door and I suddenly realize that the external door has windows out onto the street. I spend several minutes knocking progressively louder, while my naked body is visible to the passing public and beyond.

'Josie? Josie?! Can you let me in?! Josie??'

It's normally a quiet street, but today a large crowd of schoolchildren and parents are passing by on one of the final journeys before schools close. A disgusted mother shields her child's face, while others draw attention to me as I frantically knock with one hand and guard my anatomy with the other, exposing my rear due to lack of enough hands to shield myself with. Eventually the internal porch door opens to Josie in tears of laughter, shouting 'run away!' to the bounding Nelly, drawing more looks from outside. With Nelly now barking at a naked intruder, Josie sees how this is being misconstrued by the onlookers.

'It's OK, he's mine!'

She apologizes to me and through a *very* wide smile, states that she absolutely was *not* taking longer than usual to answer the door and was definitely *not* laughing in the living room for a minute or two before answering.

✚

25 March 2020 – 'Influencer' in hospital with coronavirus just days after posting a video of himself licking a toilet bowl'

With all the uncertainty and news reports making it difficult to know who to believe, I read an article about an influencer tongue kissing a toilet to 'prove' Covid-19 is safe. Ironically, they end up in hospital a few days later with coronavirus, plus probably several other infections. Mention this future 2020 to someone in 2019 and they'd have rolled their eyes and stopped taking you seriously. One thing that does seem to be true, though, is the news coming from Italy that proning (lying on your front) is therapeutic for Covid-19 patients. Proning allows more of the lungs to open up and potentially allows better oxygenation in these patients. It's an unusual way to see someone: we imagine them lying on their back or sat up in a hospital bed. But with this disease affecting the lungs so badly, proning provides simple and effective therapy. The results apparently can be pretty quick too, with patients' percentage oxygen saturations going from the 70s to high 90s in a matter of minutes. (High 90s–100 is the normal range: below that, there's generally something not quite right.)

✚

We start to ready ourselves for coronavirus hitting the hospital by simulating the proning procedure for practice, as we realize it will require turning patients regularly. It's easy enough to ask awake patients breathing for themselves to turn over, but for ventilated patients it needs a trained turning team and an airway doctor to make sure the breathing tube remains in the right place. The technique is to wrap the patient in sheets, so they resemble a Cornish pasty, followed by several moves that results in them facing down. Carl offers to model as the patient, clearly fancying a lie down after his battle briefing. We wrap him in the sheets, which look more like a spider's prey than Cornish pasty. He begins to look slightly uncomfortable and when we turn him onto his side he starts yelping loudly.

'AAOOOUUGH, arrrough!'

We turn back quickly, unwrapping the sheets to reveal he's taken his mahogany wooden pointer inside with him and it has jousted a sensitive area on turning. Carl catches his breath while we all keep straight faces.

'Check . . . no items are in the patient's bed beeeefore carefully moving them.'

✚

I take a couple of minutes to go through the airway checks on turning patients. Additional key points on our guidelines are turning off the ventilator (which occasionally puts you on edge) and clamping the breathing tube (always puts you on edge, essentially suffocating someone for a minute). After the pasty/spider's prey has been prepared and the tube clamped, you go through the turning fairly swiftly, followed by unclamping the tube (slight relief), and restarting the ventilator (total relief), at which point you and the patient can breathe again.

The reason why this manoeuvre puts us on edge is because we know that Covid patients are already very sick. These are not people having anaesthetic for surgery with otherwise healthy lungs, these are sick people whose bodies are at the edge of their compensatory mechanisms. The machines might be keeping their oxygen levels, heart rate and blood pressure at relatively normal numbers, but there now isn't anything left in reserve. Push them over that cliff and they fall fast.

✛

The rest of the day is a low-key battle preparation as we bring about the changes to make the new ICU, and all elective surgery is cancelled.

Our usual anaesthetic duties cease. We brace and prepare for the ICU onslaught.

In the blink of an eye, changes in hospital that would usually take months, years or never happen are suddenly happening all around us. If doctors or staff need it, it is there.

A new makeshift ICU complete with ventilators? *Done.*

Food and a fridge stocked with water daily? *For sure.*

Paying health-care staff what they're worth? *Don't push your luck.*

✚

There is camaraderie right across the hospital and everyone is pitching in regardless of job or grade. Making laminate signs, writing up guidelines, moving beds or computers. The children's ward chips in too, donating a dart board to spruce up the new, dull staff room. No – I don't know why they have a dart board (if nothing else, it will be good for cannula practice).

✚

Even the Covid-19 proofing in hospital has a 'community project' feeling. It is a world away from the high-tech facilities you see on TV or films about outbreaks. We don't have hazmat suits, and the hospital isn't equipped with secure biohazard glass doors or top-of-the-range materials for the biosecurity of an infectious disease. Our sealed-off Covid-19 ICU is simply plastic sheeting placed at the entrance and exit, with a zip down one side that frequently gets stuck, meaning you ungainly stoop low to enter. We take the resources we have and do the best we can.

Aside from Covid-19 itself, PPE is also suddenly everywhere. It's been a hot topic for those in the media. Either a lack of it, or the government's procurements not being fit for purpose. From my side, I've been fortunate not to have seen shortages, aside from some visors, which we had to start cleaning and reusing. This might be because I am in the prioritized area of ICU, or good management from the hospital. Either way, compared to reports of other areas of the NHS or care homes, we're lucky.

It's also a hot topic for staff, literally. Wearing a hat, an FFP3 mask, a gown, two sets of gloves (four gloves = four pieces of PPE according to the government) and a visor all add up to create a magnificent sweat fest.

On my first visit to see Covid-19 patients in ICU, I assume it is my nerves causing perspiration, seeing patients with this deadly disease that's ravaging the world, obsessing over every bit of PPE. I was hot with just a gown on, but now with all the gear I am properly sweating.

And then it begins. We hear from within the inner sanctum of the hospital that Covid-19 patients are coming in and soon some will be in ICU. We rush to get everything and anything we can ready. We are nervous, no one sure of what will happen, but team spirit is everywhere. As we enter the now-deserted ward that ICU are taking over, a message is left scribbled on the whiteboard.

'Good luck, ICU! Love from the Medical team'

The ICU fills up with Covid-19 patients fast and our emergency rota starts. Covered in PPE, for the first time I cross the boundary into the danger zone (or unzip the flimsy plastic sheet) and I start to drip beneath the gown. I'm embarrassed that people might see me sweating, but then I realize the gown is both sweat-causer and cover-up-er. Once inside, it is almost a psychological therapeutic moment, because aside from the PPE, medical life is going on as normal. Daily patient reviews are happening, some patients are awake, a few are on ventilators. It is, in medical terms, fairly normal.

✚

The first patient I see is in such good spirits that I completely forget about the whole seriousness of everything. Mrs Rose Frimley is a

Scottish woman in her 60s, slightly out of breath but managing to stave off mechanical ventilation.

'Oooh, look, another mask-face person. Have we met? I cannae remember?'

After introducing myself through the stifling mask, I mention my Scottish medical roots of studying in Aberdeen and we are off reminiscing about bonnie Scotland, how she was a schoolteacher in the Highlands, how we both miss it and love going back. A good chat and the anxiety of not knowing what lay in a Covid-19 ICU disappears.

What also disappears are the comforts I took for granted. You can't have a drink of water, go to the toilet or pop outside for anything without taking off and binning all the precious PPE you are wearing. You also cannot recognize anyone; everyone becomes a 'mask-face'. Patients see countless medical staff a day, but, like Rose, they often can't tell you who is who. Crucially, too, patients now cannot have visitors – one of the most important therapies in medicine, seeing loved ones, has stopped. This is the new normal.

It is our team's first run of night shifts and Worrall is off sick, so it's just me and Louisa on airway duties. As I finish reviewing patients in the bay, I hear a voice announce the turning team has arrived.

'All right, doc, any patients need flipping?' For the patients without sedation who hear this, I think their heart rates increase a little.

After only speaking to Rose yesterday, at the doctors' handover for my night shift I find she is now in a coma and on the ventilator, after her breathing became worse during the day and she was tiring. It was decided she would be turned onto her front tonight and because of the timing, this needs to happen at midnight, which the clock has just struck.

As the turning team get ready, I go to the head end of her bed, check the breathing tube and turn the oxygen up as the ICU nurse stands next to me to control the ventilator. We wait for the oxygen levels to rise. In normal people, breathing just air, they're usually 96–100 per cent. Mrs Frimley is now breathing only oxygen and sitting at just 91 per cent.

We go through the laminated checklist, and the team prepares the spider's prey. Once ready, I go through the steps and announce them out loud.

'Ventilator off, please' (slightly on edge).

I clamp the tube.

'Tube clamped' (on edge).

We turn and put Mrs Frimley into a front-crawl position worthy of an Olympic champion. I unclamp.

'Tube unclamped' (slight relief).

'Ventilator restart, please.'

The ICU nurse turns the ventilator back on. I am waiting for that wave of relief, but like the next breath from the ventilator, it never comes. I check Mrs Frimley's airway, into the darkness of her mouth. A few secretions pour out. The breathing tube hasn't come out or moved. I anxiously look at the ventilator and the ICU nurse trying to sort it out. A minute goes by that feels like an hour. We try restarting it again but nothing.

The oxygen starts to drop.

90,

89,

88.

We are on the precipice of that cliff.

'Can someone get Louisa?'

Louisa is tied up with another emergency. The only doctor available to me is an orthopaedic surgeon – a very good one, but the only bones breaking will be ribs if we need to start CPR.

✚

I keep a poker face while inside my panic begins to grow. If I was at an anaesthetic machine, I would stop the ventilator and use the manual balloon to give a few breaths. But this is ICU, and the ventilator has only two main settings – on or off. There is no bag for me to squeeze. What's more, all the tubing of the breathing circuit is sealed tight with tape to prevent coronavirus being generally sprinkled about.

✚

As the oxygen levels hit 87, I tell the team we are turning back to the original position. I clamp the tube and we quickly reposition, then unclamp.

The nurse hits 'go' on the ventilator and we all naively hope this will solve the problem. It doesn't. No air is going into Mrs Frimley's lungs.

The monitors beep and flash.

82,

81,

80.

She is dying in my hands, literally in my fucking hands, as I hold her head.

There is only one thing left to do.

'Cut the seals, open the circuit.'

I swivel round and grab a manual-breathing circuit with a balloon attached, something I can control. We attach the balloon, and I squeeze – air flows in and then out through the valve, which is pointing directly at my face. Now an unsealed circuit, each breath coming out at me is full of coronavirus and hitting the visor. Each leaves small droplets, centimetres from my mouth and nose. I am staring our world enemy right in the face. I am suddenly grateful for the visor.

The oxygen slowly comes up as I stare at the droplets. I take shallower breaths, thinking it might somehow stop any Covid-19 getting inside me.

Louisa arrives, sees me and quickly runs to the ventilator to help.

After a few minutes, we finally get it to work, reattach it to Mrs Frimley and make the decision not to turn again tonight.

✚

As I take off the PPE, every part of me is shaking. Taking it slowly, I remove the Covid-19-covered visor, the gloves and gown. I feel unclean.

'You OK?' Louisa smiles.

'I need a shower, I'll head to the on-call shower room.'

'OK, I won't tell you the stories about what happened there . . .'

'I'm dirty enough, thanks.'

I find a towel and get into the shower, but there is no shower gel or soap. I jump naked to the toilet next door and grab some hand wash from the sink, making it into a washable lather. The shower will only dribble, so I stand there with suds all over me, accomplishing at best a decent wash of my hands. I flashback to my shower that broke on my first day becoming a doctor. I abandon the wash down.

Later, at home, my adrenaline levels start to tail off, but I still feel unclean. I strip in the air lock, go straight into a proper shower and scrub hard, then sit down with the water flowing around me. I hope none of the coronavirus got past the visor, past the mask. I breathe more easily as it gradually washes off my hair, my face, my skin.

What won't wash is the memory of being moments away from someone dying in my hands. Someone so weakened by a virus that left them on the edge, a virus that wanted to leave the killer blow to me. Someone who just a day ago was listening to me talk about deep-fried Mars bars.

Chapter 10

Had that happened, I don't know how I'd have reacted or coped. Both patients and us live on a precipice.

✚

Nelly pops in through the open bathroom door and tilts her head at me. Stormy follows her in and sits in the doorway. Peanut then jumps into the shower from the window.

They look at me as I stare at water disappearing into the plughole. Maybe they know something is wrong, or maybe they just want feeding.

Terror mixed with relief is a potent cocktail.

I sober up a little, glad it's over.

But it is just the start.

Chapter 11

I don't think anyone was ready.

What seemed like an age of preparing disappears in an instant. The whole hospital is filled with Covid-19 patients, a tidal wave of coronavirus crashing into the wards, and we are all submerged and drowning under the force of it. At every handover, whether night or day, the team finishing the shift look ghostly and stricken. Days off feel like days on, with unavoidable exhaustion and malaise adding to your fragile mental state and bringing with it paranoia.

Is this a lack of sleep, food and constant tension?

Or have I got Covid?

＋

My self-imposed rule of not-touching-my-face-at-work is tested to the extreme at every morning handover. After scoffing a complimentary two-sausage bap, courtesy of the hospital Covid powers that be, some ketchup spurts all over the left side of my cheek. I don't have any napkins, so I wait for the handover to end with ketchup all over my face. Worrall is being his usual annoying self, pointing at me, as if I don't know it looks like someone's arterial contents have gushed all over my face.

'I know,' I keep whispering across the auditorium.

'Why are you here?' he gesticulates.

What a prick. We're all suffering with impostor syndrome, there's no need to hammer it home.

'Everything all right, guys? Anything to share?' Carl asks, in a very 'can the children at the back stop talking' tone. Everyone turns to look.

'I don't think Ed needs to be here . . . '

You utter *utter* . . .

' . . . the rota says he's off today.'

What? I check. Worrall's right, I *am* off. I've been up since 5.30am, because I have to shave each day too now, since the masks we wear for ICU supposedly only work without facial hair. Not only does this mean the death of hipsters in hospital, but it's also highly upsetting for Josie.

'You look like a child,' she grimaces. 'Maybe we should socially distance until you grow it back?'

Fuck. FUCK. FUCKKKK.

I grab my bag and slink down the steps to the front to leave.

'Ed, you've got some . . . is it blood? On your . . . '

'Yes, it is, Carl. I just murdered a sausage bap.'

On the drive home, an endorphin rush hits me about being off, and the subsequent productive day I might have. Maybe I can plant some vegetables in case of a food shortage? Or finally fix the bedroom blind so we don't wake up with the first crack of sunshine hitting the quiet world. I get in and sit down on the sofa to consider what I need for the tasks ahead of me, but soon fall asleep, waking up hours later to Nelly licking leftover traces of ketchup off my face.

✚

I look for anything to give me the slightest glimmer of escape, but it is nigh on impossible to avoid the doom. The news becomes death porn, with reports now focusing on numbers, not people. Even friends and family can't stop asking me how many people have died at work. It is the national psyche. Yes, people are dying, but you don't need to ask me. You are more likely to get news reports of places where people *didn't* die. I take to running miles and miles, over ever more weird and wonderful routes and muddy trails, anything away from my phone or the TV and my mind.

What people aren't interested in is the *slog* of days, weeks and months of tirelessly trying to keep someone alive, to suddenly fail, and how hard that is. That everything we try and do ultimately does not work. The immediacy of seeing results after treatment; the fluids, pain relief, blood, oxygen and reassurance used to bring us swift results. Now, despite everything we try, in intensive care people either make hardly any recovery or none at all.

✚

Speaking of poor results, the NHS IT system was having to work hard with updates to almost everything. Just before morning handover, I order a chest X-ray for a patient and an alert pops up.

Does this patient have a CONFIRMED case of Covid-19?

I click 'Yes'.

Do you SUSPECT this patient to have Covid-19?

Oh, I DUNNOOO . . . What happens if I click 'No'? Does the computer self-combust? Or do I?

We are embracing new technology, too, by having an app, although an app for something that works both on a personal device and an NHS computer feels like travelling back to medieval times and showing off your smartphone. It doesn't really work and nor does the system. We discover this with the new patient list app, which allows the ICU patients to be updated across the hospital and also on smartphones. There's a discharge function that would occasionally label people as dead in error. The only way of knowing was to click on the patient and see if someone had typed 'NOT DEAD' at the top.

✚

The ward round, where the team reviews each patient, now starts with us all scrambling to get PPE on first, an experience not dissimilar to school swimming trips: a cramped changing room where I try to find my goggles. As we walk into the makeshift anteroom, we're greeted by floor-to-ceiling hanging visors, as shortages have resulted in people washing and reusing them and also writing on their names, creating what looks like a memorial wall every time you enter. I make this observation and Worrall grabs my visor off the wall.

'Patrick . . .' he says in a sombre tone, '. . . gone too soon.'

I pick up his.

'Worrall . . . sadly still with us.'

✚

Out of all the stuff we wear, the gowns feel the least effective.

They're not gowns designed for dealing with an infectious disease, they're made out of what appears to be my shower curtain from university. Not watertight, and your neck and hair are pretty much exposed and left vulnerable.

On entering the 'red zone', the area where all patients have coronavirus, we first go to review Rose Frimley, the patient who we ran into trouble proning the other night. She is still unconscious on a ventilator, but her lungs look to be improving and she's needing less oxygen. With every patient we see in the unit, their problems become a replica of the last, each one suffering the effects of coronavirus, with some doing worse than others.

Ward rounds invariably take a long time in ICU, as each body system is reviewed in meticulous detail. How are the lungs, how difficult is it to ventilate? What are the oxygen levels? Is the heart struggling? Are the blood pressure and heart rate stable? Are they needing medications to support their heart? How are their kidneys? How much are they peeing? How much fluid is going in and how much is going out? The extensive list goes on and on as we keep them hovering in this half-alive, half-assisted state, from blood-sugar levels, to infection markers and antibiotics, electrolyte levels, etc. Through this meticulous tinkering, we are hoping we can optimize their path out of ICU and into the less intensive-care parts of the hospital.

✚

The ward round takes six hours. Six hours in full PPE and my body feels like it's reverted to a primordial soup. Louisa, Worrall and I all burst into the doctors' room, exhausted. It's a small, dated space with a computer and telephone on a tired desk, next to a faded sofa with some cushions the last night-shift doctors managed to commandeer. A fusty smell constantly hangs in the air and various food packaging and mugs are scattered across surfaces, the carcasses of sustenance demolished as quickly as humanly possible. The room is cluttered with unnecessary ICU paraphernalia, dusty old files and old hoarded equipment, while a few chairs take up the rest of the space. We all sink into the chairs and I open the window to give us some ventilation of our own. A joyless room, Marie Kondo would strip it bare. Just as we collapse in sweaty heaps, the phone goes from inside the red zone.

'Hi, doctor, will you do the central line on bed nine soon?'

'I . . . um wull . . . beeaa . . . wight therr,' I muffle down the phone while guzzling water and scoffing the last of a pastry, which flakes onto the phone.

✚

The central line that the caller has requested of me is a line that goes into a large vein most commonly in the neck or leg, through which medications and fluid can be given. It's generally needed in sick people in ICU. It needs ultrasound, which gives you an image of the blood vessels, tissue and where your needle is, plus it's a sterile procedure, so takes longer than putting a quick cannula in. A quick wee, sip of water and I'm already back re-donning the PPE to go in.

I scan the unit. We've taken to writing our names on our gowns too, since trying to work out who someone is from their eyes alone is difficult. It's a good idea, but today *everyone* inside the red zone is called Alex.

Raphael, a 69-year-old man, is in need of the central line. I bump into his nurse as I arrive, who, you guessed it, is called Alex.

'Ohh, you're going to do the central line? I've told him about it.'

Raphael is only lightly sedated but still has a breathing tube in his windpipe. He greets me with a slow thumbs up, as the tube entering his mouth mists and clears with every breath the ventilator helps him take. He sports a full head of hair, greyed and loosely brushed to one side, and stubble adorns his chin and face. Despite not being able to talk, his eyes and brows animate for him. I explain what needs to be done.

'So I've got to put this line into your neck, it might be a bit uncomfortable, but I'll be generous with the local anaesthetic at the start so you don't feel much?'

Another thumbs up.

I look for all the bits and pieces I need, sterile gown and gloves, central line set, ultrasound machine. Half the trouble is finding everything, but one of the Alexi has found the ultrasound machine. I look for somewhere to plug it in, but there's a spaghetti stream of wires around all the plug sockets I can see.

'Alex, can I unplug this one?' I point to the wall.

'Sure. As long as it's not the ventilator.'

Raphael raises his eyebrows and gives another thumbs up when the switch of plugs is successful and he's still breathing.

Once plugged in, I start cleaning my already gloved hands, then put on the sterile gown and another set of gloves, so now I'm wearing *three* pairs of gloves and *two* gowns, like I'm at the airport trying to get away with just hand luggage. I can't really feel anything in my fingers and my dexterity is impaired. Having not done this procedure too many times, it isn't ideal feeling less coordinated while armed with a needle and scalpel.

I start cleaning the right side of his neck with some sticks that have a sponge on the end where bright orange cleaning solution comes out, then I stick on the blue sterile drape to keep the area clean.

'Slight prick, as in just some local anaesthetic; I'm not describing myself.'

Once ready, the ultrasound machine I'm using to scan his neck breaks. In front of my and Raphael's eyes, the screen goes completely blank.

As I'm fully sterile and can't touch anything, I'm pretty helpless right now. So, Alex does all the technical NHS troubleshooting, which involves turning it off and on and checking all cables are plugged in.

'No . . . not working, we'll have to get one from the other side of the hospital.' Alex goes off to make a call.

I stand for 20 minutes, dripping on the inside of the inner gown while my hands start to wrinkle, trying not to touch anything. Since we're stuck together, I chat to Raphael, reassuring him and also commenting on the weather. I notice a family photo on the table. I keep up my inane monologue, all the while thinking of

Raphael's family who cannot see him and who he must need more than ever right now. Therapy and motivation are given by seeing people you care about, it's one of the more powerful medicines at our disposal, yet we can't use it when we most need it.

✚

Finally, another ultrasound machine arrives and Alex plugs it in. A cool blob of jelly is placed onto Raphael's neck and I use the probe to find the vessel I'm looking for. His internal jugular vein pops into view on the black-and-white screen – a white line surrounds a dark circle telling me it's the large vein I'm looking for.

'Bit of pressing now.'

I push the probe into his neck and the vein collapses; next to it another vessel doesn't and pulses away. This tells me that's his carotid artery, important because I don't want to be sticking anything in a major artery.

I take the needle and push it into his neck, watching the screen as the needle flashes into view under his skin. There's a risk of puncturing a lung, so it's always a tense moment, especially when someone's lungs are already struggling. I pull back on the syringe as the large needle heads towards the vessel. On the screen I see it enter the vein and look back at the syringe, which is filling with dark blood. Bingo. Next a long, flimsy guidewire goes through the needle into the vein, then out comes the needle altogether, leaving the wire poking out the skin from his neck. I look at the monitor as the wire can enter the heart and cause a few funny beats if it jousts around the heart chambers, but we are all clear. I take the scalpel and make a cut next to the wire, hoping that I don't drop it from my three-gloved grasp and lacerate his neck open. Dark blood rolls out and I try to mop it up with a swab; Alex shakes her head at me as I make a bloody mess everywhere. Eventually everything is ready and I pass the central line (basically a big plastic tube) over the wire, through his skin, sliding it easily into his internal jugular vein, and remove the guidewire. It needs to be stitched in, which is one of my least pretty skills, so I haphazardly tie up threads with some rudimentary knots, not too dissimilar to my shoelace efforts when at primary school. Hopefully no one is watching me.

'Is that what you call a *stitch*?'

Of course, Worrall is watching. I offer him the opportunity to finish the knots, but he suddenly has something else to do.

Finally, I tear off the sterile gown and third pair of gloves, trying not to damage the ones underneath, and immediately feel some relief from the heat.

'All done, Raphael.'

He smiles, then taps the bed to get my attention. He holds his hands and gesticulates writing on paper, like signing for a bill in a restaurant.

'Oh, no no, don't worry, we're not in America. No bills this time.'

He smiles, and tries to laugh, with difficulty as he has a breathing tube in. He gesticulates again and I realize he literally means a pen and paper. So I pass him both and he scrawls something, then hands it back to me.

Thank you, it says.

'Oh, no problem, really it's my job. I've just been a pain in the neck to you, well, if it wasn't for the local anaesthetic.'

Off comes all the PPE again and it feels like jumping into the sea as a breeze hits my wet face. I'm sick of this claustrophobic gear. I hang my visor on the remembrance wall and head back to the doctors' office. The phone rings.

'Oh, Ed, central line for bed 11, please.'

No rest. No let up. No end in sight.

✚

Over the rest of the day Raphael gives me a wave each time I pass him in the red zone. As the unit continues to fill with patients, he's to be transferred to another hospital with more space than us, as he is fortunately less sick than others here. I start getting his notes and things ready, then take him to the red-zone door and wave him off as the transfer team collect him. I hope he makes it.

✚

My bleep goes off and it's Louisa on the medical ward.

'We've got another patient not doing well who's just coming in, we'll have to tube.'

Sarika arrives, our new patient, in her early 40s, who up until recently has been coping on the ward with CPAP (continuous positive airway pressure, basically a tight-fitting mask that helps with breathing). Now, though, she's struggling with her breathing so much that she needs to be intubated before she gets even more tired and unwell. She's sweating and restless, drenched dark hair strands drape over her face and the uncomfortable mask she wears. We chat through what needs to happen but it's not ideal. I have to shout because of the mask I have on, but also because of the mask Sarika has on.

'Do you want me to call anyone?'

'My mum.'

I call her mum while at the bedside and talk/shout through what is going to happen.

Chapter 11

Then I place the phone close to Sarika's head and help communicate.

'I love you,' her mum says, but Sarika can't hear so I try to help.

'I. LOVE. YOU.'

She smiles and between breaths says:

'Oh . . . well . . . that's very . . . nice of you, doctor, I'm . . . flattered. I . . . am . . . single . . . you . . . know.'

'Oh no, I MEAN YOUR MUM!'

'I . . . know . . . I'm . . . joking . . . Tell her . . . I . . . love her too . . .'

I relay the message.

Suddenly she looks at me and says:

'Is this . . . the . . . right . . . thing . . . to do?'

I look at her oxygen levels, only 82 per cent on pure oxygen, her breathing rapid and looking tired.

The answer before Covid was always easy: *yes, this is the right thing*, but now it's grey. If we don't intubate she will probably die, but if we do she might die anyway. I look open-mouthed behind my mask.

'This is the right thing,' Louisa assures her. 'You're not going to be able to breathe much longer without this, it's the only way we can take care of you.'

'O . . . K,' she says.

Louisa and I get everything ready for intubation. The controlled environment of an anaesthetic room, with a single patient in a calm atmosphere, is long gone. That seems a world away on this open ward.

'See . . . you . . . soon,' Sarika says.

Louisa checks that we're all ready and we start. I inject the anaesthetic drugs in quick succession, since Sarika's oxygen levels are so low we need to do this as fast as possible. After a minute, Louisa places the laryngoscope in Sarika's mouth and quickly places the tube. We connect up to a ventilator and soon her breaths are all coming from the machine, the animation and wit Sarika showed just moments ago gone.

That's the difference between this disease and others. People are still *with it* despite being critically unwell, they keep their faculties about them. Still able to share jokes in their own moments of darkness, but also to cognitively question if it's the right thing. I think of Raphael and Sarika over the coming days. Hamish was right, it's *always* about the patients. I wonder how Raphael is getting on. I always stop by to check on Sarika.

✚

Until one day, she's no longer there.

Chapter 12

There have been so many Covid-19 patients that I've never had a conversation with, and still I know their faces and medical needs better than many of the patients I've been lucky enough to speak to over my career.

Many come to the unit unwell and need to be put into an induced coma, after which they either stay ventilated for a very long time, or die, with the resulting bedspace soon filled by another Covid-19 victim. Mrs Rose Frimley is still holding on. It's been over a month now and, as one of the last patients I had a conversation with, for some reason I feel a lot rests on her recovery.

In fact, ventilated patients in ICU are pretty much all I've seen for such a long time. In my head I try to imagine what patients are like when they're awake. Those with pictures by their beds allow me a glimpse of smiles and family life. I imagine how they speak, the expressions they pull, the jokes they make, what they look like when they laugh or are surprised, if they're loud or quiet and reserved. I want to understand them as people and not just patients as they lie here in purgatory. In anaesthetics people could also be ventilated for a long time, but you'd meet them before the operation and again after the surgeon (finally) finishes. I miss the people behind the stats we check through every day, I miss the human who has been taken out of this body as it tries to survive and we try and stop it from dying.

✚

Mr Luke Kim on the unit is one such patient I've not met before and he needs a CT (computed tomography) scan. It's a common scan, and you may have even had one yourself. In normal times getting to a scan appointment is simply walking in, lying on the bed and getting whirred into the CT machine, which looks like a giant Polo. Even if you can't walk, you can be brought down in a chair or bed, maybe by a porter or nurse, then more kind people will help you across to the scanner. When people can't walk *and* can't breathe, the journey is a bit more fraught.

Luke needs a CT scan on his lungs to check for clots, one of the side effects of having this infection. Since he's got a breathing tube in and a ventilator is breathing for him, it would be *slightly* unfair to leave this to the porter, not that any are free. He's also got a central line, arterial line (to measure blood pressure direct from his artery), a urinary catheter, a nasogastric tube (for feeding, which goes into his stomach via his nose), plus other drips/drugs and monitoring. So, there's a bit of luggage in tow.

Jacob, his nurse, and I will be doing taxi duties. I want to tell you transferring a ventilated patient is a nice smooth process, the press of a button and things set in motion, automatically you enter cruise control. The reality is much more basic, likened to pushing two or three full trolleys around a supermarket with a couple of upright mops sticking out. A supermarket is probably better, as the aisles are wider.

We start getting everything ready and go through a transfer checklist to ensure we don't miss anything. I prepare emergency drugs in case Luke becomes even more unwell on the journey, Jacob fetches spare oxygen cylinders, a spare battery for the ventilator, and we pack everything we need for the trip. We also stow his drug infusions on the bed for the journey, the pumps containing propofol, a muscle relaxant and strong opiate.

A transfer of this type is an obstacle course, with hazards such as tubes and lines getting caught, or doors shutting on the bed and you. One of the worst things to happen is something catching the breathing tube and pulling it out of Luke's mouth, hence it needs an airway doctor to go along, to troubleshoot any issues like that. Although putting a Covid breathing tube in mid-corridor while the general public stand around open-mouthed holding coffee is not a situation I'd *ever* want to be in. I can imagine some people looking aghast, while others carry on as normal at the till.

'A cappuccino and americano, please. Oh, and anything for you, doctor?'

'Quick, the VENTILATOR!' I'd yell.

'He'd like a venti latte, please.'

✚

Once ready, I push the head end so I'm close to any tube issues. The brakes come off the bed and we creep forward, while I hook the ventilator with my arms to roll with the bed and me. We start our way through the unit, passing other unconscious patients tended to by ICU nurses, the heart and soul of ICU. No ICU can function without these valuable and specialized nurses. As doctors, we look after all patients, but nurses intimately know individual patients and their ongoing progress and story, without which we couldn't do our job.

✚

It's not long before we're cursing the hospital's haphazard structure once more, finding it far too narrow once we are outside the unit. We become wedged between the red-zone exit and the narrow corridor wall. People come to temporarily clear the clutter, boxes and trolleys that have nowhere else to go, then there's a slow-motion comedy of forwards and backwards a few times just to turn the corner, in order to leave the ICU.

'Argggh!' Jacob yells, then disappears to the floor beyond my sight.

'Shit, Jacob? Are you OK?'

'Yeah . . . ' He stands gingerly. 'I just stood on my scrubs and tripped myself up.'

He dusts himself down and we finally have space to turn the corner. Even if you wanted to improve this place, the hospital is plagued with a history of asbestos, so even the most minor work becomes a health and safety nightmare. It really needs to be knocked down, but then it can't be, because of said asbestos. A perfect and awful excuse. It's one of the most frustrating things. I want to give people the best care in the best place, but we end up with patched-up buildings held together by gaffer tape.

Jacob, Luke and I bump along the uneven corridor floor.

'Wait wait wait!'

I shout, seeing the tubing from the ventilator attached to Mr Kim's breathing tube catch on a door handle and begin to stretch. I unhook it and pull the ventilator close, kicking away some more boxes.

'OK, off we go again.'

A supermarket *is* better than this.

Once outside, it feels like an escape from the unit, back into normal hospital land. The background noise of ICU monitors beeping and chatter slowly disappears as we exit. We're away from the unit now, outside.

My life has been in Covid ICU so much that I have rarely seen the rest of the hospital, with my work focused inside the unit. Outside, other areas of hospital are quieter or shut. We move slowly, past the quieter than usual operating theatres, where I suddenly have a pang of yearning. That's where I used to anaesthetize and feel excited, *home*. One positive bit of news is that dexamethasone (or dex, as it's known in the hospital corridors) has been found to be a treatment for Covid patients needing oxygen. It's fantastic and also nostalgic. Matt Hancock (the then-government Health Secretary) talks as if he has just invented it out of thin air, like he personally just discovered penicillin, but dex is an old, old drug. Dex has been used for decades as an anti-sickness medication by anaesthetists; midwives and obstetricians give it to women who are at risk of pre-term labour to help develop their babies' lungs, and also as a treatment for croup (the barking cough children can get). I would rarely go a day without using it. In anaesthetics, you always give dex after the patient is asleep, as a side effect is an itchy perineum. An itchy gooch can be pretty uncomfortable for anyone, more so for patients already nervous and trying to keep a straight face for their operation.

✚

On we go, past some vending machines selling cans and snacks, while through my mask I can smell the canteen baked potatoes and beans from down the corridor. I'd just love it if we could stop here, me, Jacob and Luke, grab a cold drink, talk about the good old pre-Covid days.

As we roll, I wonder if Luke somehow knows we're outside the unit, and whether it's a therapeutic change?

Occasionally people stare as we roll past, horrified that someone has a tube in their mouth and a ventilator in tow. A sight of the inner sanctum of Covid that all news channels are reporting about, us dressed in full PPE. People's chatter hushes as they see us arrive and compute where we've come from. The monitor's beeps are the only noises left in the corridor – the reassuring bustle of active corridors, people talking and catching up now gone, the traffic less, same as the roads.

I spot Sally down the corridor and get excited. She must be the consultant anaesthetist on emergency theatres today. Sally stops to let us pass.

'Hi, Sally!' I shout with a wave. She waves back but clearly doesn't recognize me behind the mask and gear. She moves along towards theatres.

We pass the pre-op clinic, shut because of Covid, while the backlog of patients needing surgery mounts.

My family, like many others, have been hit. Not long ago, I joined Dad at a pre-op appointment back home, for an operation to remove a cancer. I remember the tense conversation.

'The results say highly suspicious of cancer. It needs to come out,' the consultant asserts to me.

'*Suspicious*, not definitely cancer then? Surely there's another way?' I plead, knowing Dad is high risk for any surgery now.

The consultant sighs, losing his patience with me. Dad has been referred for surgery and the surgeon just wants to do his job, not think outside the box. There is pressure for a decision to have the operation before surgery shuts down in a couple of weeks because of the Covid wave. It would be incredibly high risk, with a high chance of never being himself afterwards, or dying.

Do we take a high risk of death? Or chance a potential cancer that might also kill? We chance it. Dad says no, against the surgeon's advice.

I also suspected that when Covid hit and the hospitals filled, if Dad needed an ICU bed he wouldn't get one. On our unit he'd have struggled to: everyone here is younger than him. It isn't just here. Every ICU in the country is filling with younger patients. If there's only one bed and two people need it, it will go to the person most likely to make a recovery. With Dad's heart condition, he wouldn't even be a candidate. As we walk through these deserted corridors, I wonder whether we've made the right decision. Time will tell.

I should add that Luke, Jacob and I are Covid-safe in the corridor because we're not touching anything and all the breathing circuits are closed, but there is literally no other way to get to the scanner anyway. We turn the final corner and see the open doors to CT.

'Come in,' the radiographer beckons.

In another great design feature of this hospital, there's a downhill camber just as you head towards the CT doors, so you need to time exactly when you hit the slope so that the momentum takes you into the scanner room. The alternative is rolling down the hill and smashing through the window at the end into the car park. Which would be a nightmare, as the parking attendants are ruthless.

Just as we time our move onto the camber, the radiographer pops out again.

'Oh, actually, wait, please! Just a couple of minutes.'

I see Jacob's eyes and forehead go from concentrated neutral to almost red with the effort of stopping us from rolling downhill. I brace the bed and the ventilator from the top end. One side of the ventilator wheels rises up slightly, the oxygen cylinders rattle around, Luke shakes from side to side. Our feet grip and give as we try to stop the bed. Eventually we come to a stop and turn sideways and we hit the brakes, Jacob still bracing.

'Are you OK?' I ask him

'Yeah, and Luke's oxygen levels have gone up to 93 per cent.'

'Fantastic, we'll tilt him to this side when we get back then.'

Patients with Covid seem to have a good side that you lean them towards, and we've just found Mr Kim's.

I look behind me and see the entrance to the maternity centre, the place I met Josie for the first time. If we met now, we wouldn't even see each other's faces.

Chapter 12

✚

'We're out of oxygen.'

I turn back slightly wide-eyed at Jacob's announcement.

'Just changing it across to the next,' he follows up.

'I thought you were about to tell me we'd forgotten to bring the oxygen.'

Still, that's 460 litres of oxygen gone in a frighteningly short space of time. I thought it was the one thing that would always be in plentiful supply at hospitals, pre-Covid. When I started anaesthetics, all newbies attended a simulation course, which was a mixture of lectures dotted with snippets of tales such as thiopentone, an old anaesthetic drug that may have been responsible for killing more American soldiers at Pearl Harbor than those fighting.

The rest was simulations, designed to run you through stressful situations, so that in real life you wouldn't act like a deer in headlights about to shit yourself. Everyone has to tackle a scenario, which is filmed and screened to everyone else sitting next door, like some low-key reality game show.

When my turn comes, I'm waiting for something to go wrong because it has to. The patient in bed is a full-sized, body mannequin that can blink, talk and breathe. I have an assistant who strangely doesn't talk much but will fetch things. Full of tension, I try not to muck up the scenario in front of everyone in the room, behind the one-way mirror and those watching on TV next door, plus the mannequin.

My brain scrambles over what's going to happen. Will they become unconscious and require intubation? Go into cardiac arrest? Have they been in a house fire or road traffic accident?

My scenario unexpectedly and ironically turns out to be a failed oxygen supply to the hospital. I fumble around and fetch some oxygen cylinders and generally made sure no one dies, but I remember thinking *what a completely bonkers scenario*. Surely that won't happen in a UK hospital? Yet among the deluge of warnings we get daily, one is that the hospital is indeed struggling with oxygen supply.

✚

'OK, you can come in now.' The radiographer's head pops out again.

Jacob and I push hard to get the bed going uphill slightly, then turn into the scanner room. Once inside, we transfer Luke to the scanner bed. His oxygen levels immediately drop to 87 per cent, so we move swiftly to get the scan done. Drug pumps, tubing, lines, ventilator, drips all moved across, then the radiographer does a test run with the bed moving in and out of the scanner, to make sure there's no tugging on tubes or lines. Once ready, we pop out the room and I watch his vital signs through the glass as the scanner gets to work.

Breathe in says the automated voice to an unconscious patient.

We wait as the scan does its thing, taking a couple of minutes, and watch as his oxygen levels continue hovering.

'OK, all done!'

We go back in and transfer Luke back to the bed, then move on out, hitting the camber again.

'His oxygen is up to 92 per cent again!' Jacob announces.

'Maybe we just park here? Seems the best place.'

We decide against leaving Luke there and instead head back to the unit, moving through the hospital, breathing heavily through the tight masks from the exercise.

✚

Once we arrive back into the ICU ecosystem, my bleep goes off inside and it's Louisa.

'Ed . . . ah, ah . . . Ed?' The sound of Louisa slightly unable to talk.

'Yeah, it's Ed. Is that you, Louisa? Are you OK?'

'Yeah ... fine, ah ... ah ... ' I hear the sound of a gulp. 'Sorry, I was eating a Mars bar and downing a Coke, starving! I didn't expect you to answer so quickly. Could you pull back Mrs Frimley's tube? Looks like it's slipped down a bit on her recent scan.'

If a breathing tube slips down, the anatomy means it will migrate towards your right lung, which then gets all the breaths and pressure, whereas the left is bypassed. It can lead to complications, such as trauma caused by overpressure to the right lung, so we want it at a level where both lungs are working together.

Mrs Rose Frimley is in a coma still, but out of courtesy I introduce myself and explain what I'm about to do.

'Hi, Rose, it's Ed the doctor, we spoke about Scotland and a few other things a while back.'

Her eyes are closed, her artificial breaths the only movement.

'So, the breathing tube in your mouth is a little lower than we'd like, so I'm just going to pull it back a bit.'

I go around to her head, and step over cables and wires to get there. Her face is relaxed, eyes shut, mouth ajar with the tube protruding. Her body only moves in rhythm to the ventilator with each breath it delivers. Wires from various monitoring cross her torso.

'Ah ah ah, doctorrr.'

Chapter 12

Maria, the ICU nurse, rolls the 'rr' at the end of 'doctor' accusingly at me and wags a finger.

'I've just washed and combed her hair, don't you dare go and disturb that.'

'Maria, I daren't risk my life disturbing your handiwork.'

She laughs and hands me a stethoscope hanging nearby.

'Here, it's clean but obviously we're inside a Covid ward and . . . well, as clean as it can be.'

'Don't worry, I'm not going to lick my ears,' I say, popping the tight, plastic and downright uncomfortable earpieces into my ears.

I have a listen to Rose's chest, and note the quiet breath sounds from the right side compared to the left, so I undo the ties holding the breathing tube and pull it back, then re-listen. Her ventilation and oxygen levels improve slightly too.

'All sounds good, Rose. My work is done here. I'll escape before Maria scolds me again.'

✚

At the end of handover, I'm in the changing room alone as it's so late. I pull off scrubs and throw them into the overflowing plastic bag in the corner. It's Sunday, I'm starving, with nowhere open, and Josie is on a night shift. Maybe we've got some beans? If not, it's cat food for tea. My phone buzzes and there's an email sent to all doctors in hospital.

Food and drink on A&E today!

Yes! Hospital managers have treated us to some food. Teamwork and supporting each other. It's the one thing that's kept us going through all this. There are lots of problems that need addressing in the NHS, but right here, right now the things that make a difference are human. The acts of kindness, conversation, connection and food.

I wander down to A&E, wondering who I might see and what food they've planned for us. I arrive to a fairly deserted department, a few doctors and nurses mingling about, no one putting out food, indeed no one has heard anything about this generous offering. In the staff room there's nothing, just one person with a cup of tea. I check my phone. Had I imagined the email? No, it's there. I read the rest of it.

Re: Food and Drink on A&E today!
This is a notice to all staff. Please can you refrain from eating or drinking anywhere in A&E.

Chapter 13

Several of us, many more than necessary, are assisting this special transfer of a patient.

Louisa and Worrall are either side of the bed, guiding it through the doorway from ICU, as the rest of us file out behind them. We coast along the hot corridors, because despite it being 25°C (77°F) outside, in classic hospital fashion the heating is on and no one knows how to turn it off. The hospital feels busier than usual too, with more people around, many of whom are reluctantly standing with their backs pressed up against hot radiators in order to let our entourage pass. We move faster than normal for an ICU transfer and the bed feels lighter as there's no ventilator or drug pumps. Onwards we go, turning into the CT scanner corridor, except that's not where we're going. We hit the downhill camber, but instead of going into the scanner room, or braking to prevent us flying out of the hospital, we continue towards the glass window, turn into the doorway and out of the hospital. A great escape.

All of us are wearing masks, but in our eyes we're smiling. Passers-by stare as, unconventionally, medical staff with a patient in tow exit the hospital and head out into the sun. The sun hits our blue scrubs, probably the first natural light they've ever seen. This request for natural vitamin D came from the patient we are escorting, which was prescribed by the consultant and duly administered by us. I've no idea if it was ever OK'd by hospital management to bring a patient outside: none of us asked the question, expecting the answer would be negative. But then again it never made sense what *was* and *wasn't* allowed. Pre-pandemic, I was once scolded for carrying a disposable coffee cup because of potential infection-control issues. Later that same evening, I watched a news report about a hospital bringing a horse inside to raise patient morale.

'Ahhhh,' Rose Frimley sighs, as she turns her palms up towards the sun.

Rose, after several months in ICU, has both cleared her coronavirus infection and isn't far from being discharged back to the ward, then hopefully home. She basks in the sun. Her mouth, no longer occupied by a breathing tube, works into a smile revealing her teeth as she takes deep breaths of her own making. A piña colada and sunglasses short of being on a sunbed in Mexico.

Chapter 13

'Well, it's certainly warmer than Scotland,' Rose remarks, shielding her eyes.

'It certainly is,' I agree and retell the time ice formed inside my Aberdeen bedroom one morning, then in the evening the roof leaked with rainwater, all of which failed to impress the landlord enough to do anything.

'I was living in my own glen,' I tell her.

Here, it is an escape for all of us.

A celebration that a long-term Covid patient has finally pulled through. Our efforts have paid off. We all bask in the sunlight together, collectively appreciating the moment in reverential silence.

Then, a parking attendant interrupts us as he instinctively grabs his ticket machine at the sight of something with four wheels near a double yellow line, but upon seeing us he resists the urge.

✚

There was no exact turning-point when things started to get better. As with all things in life, there wasn't a big moment where everything was suddenly resolved, but gradually patient numbers started to settle, the wave began to die down, the patients less so.

Gradually, we had beds staying empty for longer and patients with medical problems other than coronavirus coming into ICU for support.

More people were leaving alive.

✛

'Shall we go to the roof?' Hans, the ICU consultant, asks.

We all look at each other with frowns of surprise, because for the first time in ages all the patients are stable and we realize we don't need to keep a constant vigil.

'Let's go.' Hans leads us out.

We head up a rickety, metal staircase through a security door, into an area of the hospital I've never been to before. As we go across the roof, we can see the swarm of hospital below us. In one corner of the roof there are some old, dusty plastic patio chairs arranged in a circle, plus a table and some detritus of old food and drinks lying about. Louisa, Worrall, me, some first-year doctors and a few surgeons all brush the chairs down and sit, heads up to the sky – letting a moment of normality sink into our addled bodies. No mention of ICU or Covid. Twenty minutes goes past as we collectively catch our breath. We all silently breathe, deeply, replenishing and filling ourselves up before heading back inside to exhale.

Inside, patients still need us, still need the oxygen, the pipes running deep through the walls and ceilings of the hospital to individual ports that connect to patients. The coffee shop continues to feed caffeine to the workforce. Colleagues continue to overheat and exhaust themselves in ICU and across the hospital. The mortuary, I hope, is less busy.

✚

And then, simultaneously, all our phones buzz with a notification. An email to everyone saying that coronavirus cases are settling, redeployment will soon end. The end of the emergency rota, meaning this red team would be no more. And there it is, happiness, but also a sense of sadness descends on all of us, for everything we've been through. No longer a team. I won't see Louisa, or, dare I say it, even Worrall, on a regular basis.

✚

There isn't really anything to show for our collective struggle. No special mention, no particular recognition other than the odd email or letter to say thanks and farewell. The hospital gradually creaks open other services and clinics, hurriedly trying to deal with the backlogs.

✚

The joy I hotly anticipated of this, let's be honest, pretty fucking momentous moment of Covid-19 not controlling everything never appears.

✚

I'm just numb with exhaustion, both mentally and physically.

✚

I thought the end would bring jubilation, but it's more of a moment to catch your breath after the long uphill run and now relative unease. Because everything and everyone worth listening to points to another wave, another battle. This is only a respite. On my phone, I open up a news bulletin from the Royal College of Anaesthetists (RCOA) and see an article.

RCOA calls for anaesthetists to take holiday in preparation for Covid second wave

The title says it all. Anaesthetists are being told to relax while holding the brace position. And all this while engaging with the worry of ongoing job admin – getting enough anaesthetics experience to be signed off, job interviews and exams. I scroll down the newsletter but sadly cannot find a voucher entitling anaesthetists to a free, all-inclusive, beach holiday.

It brings home the reality facing us. Airway doctors are in short supply, especially in intensive care. That is partly why they need anaesthetists to work there still, but we also need this burned-out workforce with a very specific skillset to reset, and reset quickly.

What can we do?

✚

I try to relax and arrange to see my parents for the first time since the pandemic began. Dad has managed to have his appointment, for the biopsy of a suspected cancer that was due to be removed by the life-threatening operation cancelled just before the pandemic. Except it *isn't* cancer after all. What they initially thought was a sinister growth is benign, harmless. After all that – the appointments, stress, worry, the not knowing the right thing to do and moral wrangling. The operation he so nearly had, that could quite easily have killed him, wasn't needed in the first place. I think back to the moment when he cancelled and shake my head.

Sometimes the most powerful thing you can do in medicine is nothing at all.

✚

It is only Josie's second time meeting my parents and I am slightly on edge. Before the pandemic hit, Josie met my family and the memory of it is etched in my brain.

There was a big family coming together of my brother and his family, my sister and her family. It's pretty daunting meeting such a large group, but Josie was cool, calm and excited, like any good midwife always ready for the main event.

We meet at my parent's house and as we arrive everyone is already in the garden, my nieces and nephew running around as Dad brings various beverages from the fridge. I hope this intense meet and greet goes well and I relax as Josie manages to instantly get on with the children. I can already see my brother wondering if the family could adopt Josie in place of me. This feels strangely fun and warming. I pop inside for a drink, wondering why I have been worrying about this meeting for such a long time and making such a big deal of it all. Racking my brains, I can't remember *why* I ever thought my parents meeting partners was so embarrassing, it's clearly not. They're just normal parents?

I wander back outside to hear Mum asking Josie:

'So, have you ever read the *Kama Sutra*?'

Ah, *now* I remember.

If I thought that was bad, the reason for this line of questioning is in order for my mum to set up the story of when I, aged 18, bought lingerie as a gift for an ex. Having never bought something like this before, I *inexplicably* asked *my mum* for an opinion (reader, I'm sorry, I don't know why I did this, trust me).

A silence falls, pregnant with unbearable giggling tension as my family quietly try to restrain themselves, the children ask respective parents what lingerie is, while Josie wipes away tears of shocked laughter.

She's going to end our relationship after this.

Just as I was sweating from every pore at this deeply buried memory hurtling back, I nearly pass out at Mum's attempt to bring us back to a normal line of conversation.

'I mean, he's got very good taste . . .

' . . . they weren't crotchless or anything.'

I head back inside for more drinks and proceed to scream into a towel in the bathroom.

✚

I also have time to catch up with Max from medical school, now a GP. Still up in Scotland, but residing in Edinburgh. His tales of GP-land remind me of medical life outside of hospital and the other Covid syndromes, in particular his fascination with Covid toe. I've been so focused on the critically ill that I've not heard of the milder things coronavirus is causing.

'So, I've seen one Covid toe, some colleagues have seen more, though,' he says excitedly.

'What is it?'

'They're like chilblains, red patches on the toes, but they're not chilblains.'

'Right, chilblains but not chilblains,' I say, thinking I haven't spent too much time looking at toes in ICU. 'So how do you treat it?'

'You don't!' he exclaims. 'You just get to tell other people you've seen it.'

Covid toe-spotting, the new trainspotting.

✚

And gradually a sense of normal life does creep back in, but at home we keep the changes we introduced when it all began. We keep the air lock going, so used to showering after hospital now. In fact, it seems odd that we never did before. Some colleagues have even embraced the heightened infection awareness to their advantage. In the staff room sweet treats would normally disappear faster than a piece of steak set upon by piranhas. But someone, who clearly wants to have their cake and eat it, has labelled a chocolate fudge cake with:

Covid Cake, do not touch!

No one knows what it means. Is it a present from a Covid patient? Has it come from a place of Covid? The delicious cake and icing remained untouched, as passers-by stare suspiciously. Some stretch out a hand to try it, but then hold themselves back. But later on, when I pass by, it has been demolished, with only crumbs remaining and not a perpetrator in sight.

✚

I even get the chance to head back to do some anaesthetics and it is a delight. I join Dr Commons for a list one afternoon.

'You seem happy.'

'I can't tell you how happy I am to be back in theatre!'

I take his constant grumpiness towards me with the joy of knowing that today I'm an anaesthetist.

I lap up everything I've missed, being able to *talk* to patients, give drugs for an operation, work with ODPs again, seeing someone wake up and soon be back to their normal selves. I've missed giving oxygen and seeing a patient's levels reassuringly rise. I even tap the anaesthetic machine like it's an old trusty car that I have had since late adolescence.

'Did you just affectionately tell the anaesthetic machine that you *missed* it?'

I hadn't realized Dr Commons was also in the room.

I blissfully listen to the surgeon drone on and on during the operations, while taking a huge amount of pleasure in the admin of filling out an anaesthetic chart and prescribing post-operative medications for the patient.

At lunchtime, in the corridor, I bump into Louisa and we share each other's mutual joy to be back doing some anaesthetics.

'It's coming back, though. My mum has it,' Louisa says.

'Oh no, I'm so sorry to hear.'

'She's OK, thankfully, on the mend. But the infections are just going up and up,' she gesticulates with both hands above her head. 'We'll be back in Covid ICU soon, Ed.'

My mood sinks at the thought as we both pull dissatisfied faces. I look down at my belly paunch thoughtfully and back to Louisa.

'Do you think they'll give us free sausage sandwiches again?'

Chapter 14

The highly anticipated second wave does hit, and hits hard. But in addition to fear, there is a feeling of frustration on the wards. We've been through this, got it under control and now we have to down tools and do it all over again. Our government's policies and decisions haven't worked. And we have been slammed.

Everything becomes a weighted effort. The PPE for some reason feels heavier, the masks are more claustrophobic. The exhaustion from the first wave is still there, particularly mentally. Seeing so many people die in a short space of time and feeling all your effort, everything you do, unable to stop it from happening saps at everyone's energy and optimism. All my anaesthetic shifts for operations, which felt therapeutic to look at, are abandoned as they all automatically become ICU shifts again. This time, there would be no set teams. At least I don't have to work with Worrall again.

Just getting ready for work now feels cumbersome. Our schedules mean Josie and I are constantly at home at different ends of the day. I wake up to see she has left a drawer open (a little *annoying* perk of hers) and although it is Covid times and we strip in our porch, I shut it to maintain some sort of 'let's keep our house a bit more Feng Shui'. But I should have looked first, as I receive an unimpressed message from her hours later, reading:

'Stormy has been stuck in the blanket drawer ALL DAY!'

Along with a picture of said unimpressed cat, that had since been trapped in a drawer for several hours. Come to think of it, he *does* look like a rolled-up blanket. But I empathize with Stormy, as I re-enter the hospital and feel ever more enclosed by the mighty drawer-closing government that has lodged us firmly back into the second-wave drawer.

✚

I think to myself, maybe the wave won't be as bad? Maybe it will be easier?

But it's worse and the patients are getting younger.

Jack was in his 50s, he had dark short hair, and that's all I ever got to know about him. He died before our handover finished: my first job was to verify his death. Like many others, one day ago Jack came into the unit, Covid-19 positive, struggling with breathing and needing to be ventilated. Everything the ICU could do had been done, but nothing worked. He would be alive if not for coronavirus.

✚

I pull on PPE and head to the side room, unusually quiet because none of the machines are on or showing signs of life. For a minute I just stand silently, looking at Jack, the bed, the room. I speak to him, just in case and out of my routine courtesy, because I'm so used to asking permission from patients and explaining to them what I'm about to do.

'Hi, Jack, I'm just going to have a listen to your chest and feel for a . . . feel your pulse.'

I take a stethoscope and listen to his lungs, heart, looking for any signs of his chest moving. Nothing, his skin cold, a stillness in the air.

More people seem to die than survive in the unit: the second wave is relentless with death and there's little we can do to help because everyone becomes so unwell so quickly. The day in the sun with Rose, when things seemed to be getting better, seems a long way away.

When will it ever end?

✚

'Do you think Mum will be all right?'

I exhale away from the ICU telephone, under my tight-fitting mask that is making my face ache. Without exception, a pang of awfulness goes through me when people ask this. So used to using a patient's name that a mention of a family word, by people outside of this lifeless vacuum, always shakes you out of your professional comfort zone.

Son,

daughter,

mum,

dad,

auntie,

uncle.

Boyfriend,

girlfriend,

wife,

husband.

The daughter, Caroline, that I'm speaking to sounds younger than my sister, and she is asking about her mum, Lucy, who's much, much younger than my mum. This is the awful thing about the second surge, people *are* younger and many more are dying. Any progress, success or gain feels so much smaller and more marginal than before. Earlier, Maria and I altered Lucy's pillows and her oxygen saturations went up by 1 per cent, the first time they'd gone up in hours, yet because of the total lack of progress people are making, we cheered, seeing this as a win.

Nothing, for anyone, was going in the right direction.

'It doesn't look good, Caroline. I'm afraid your mum might die.'

Fucking, fucking hell.

What the FUCK am I saying?

Why am *I* saying this?

A disease I knew nothing about a year ago . . .

. . . and suddenly I'm telling people their family members are dying and we still don't

FUCKING KNOW WHY.

We've been taught to know the differences, to understand what to do when people present themselves in a certain way, we've done more multiple-choice exams than any sane person should ever have to perform. We've been told that good doctors have the right answers, but every conversation I am having has become vague, overlayed with negative forewarnings, nothing can be definitive. Nothing can be factual. Nothing works.

Is there anything else you can do, doctor?

We're doing all we can, but it might not be enough, things could change in minutes, hours or days.

How are they?

Stable for now, but critically unwell, and they might die.

When?

I can't tell you if or when, but possibly soon.

I FUCKING HATE IT ALL.

Medicine.

Medicus curat, natura sanat.

'The physician cares while nature heals.'

Where *is* the healing?

Why is it not *here*?

Why am I also suddenly proficient in Latin quotes?

✚

'Thank you for everything you're doing,' Caroline says as she finishes the call.

Guilt floods through me when she says this. Because it feels like I'm not doing anything at all.

Chapter 15

I can't remember the last time I slept well, before hospital anyway.

Tonight is no exception. Josie is on night shift, so it's just me in bed and I have woken up in a cold sweat. Then I realize I've knocked a glass of water over myself, plus the heating has broken down.

Lacking a hot water bottle, I go for the next best thing.

'Nelly??'

Little thuds start up the stairs and get louder as Nelly closes in, then jumps on the bed.

'Ugh,' I yelp as a paw lands unsympathetically in my groin.

Excited, thinking it's time for an early breakfast, Nelly is slightly surprised when she realizes the calling was for some life-saving skin-to-fur warmth. She semi-reluctantly settles under the duvet and lets out a yawn before promptly snoring on Josie's pillow. It's 3am, freezing, and I'm spooning my girlfriend's cockapoo.

Of course, I'm exhausted, which adds to the irony of not being able to sleep.

It's difficult to dissociate whether it's the physical or emotional toll causing more tiredness. The resurgence of coronavirus and ICU work has been like watching the same horror movie on repeat, but with the admin of job applications, interviews and yearly appraisal it means work creeps up and into home life, with no escape to keep it at bay.

The days off are numbing. The days on are numbing.

Just as my thoughts bore me into a slumber, my alarm goes off, so I drag myself out of bed, make an extra-strong coffee to go, then charge out of the door to hospital.

Just like people don't remember having an anaesthetic, I struggle to remember which day it is. There is no weekend, there are no days. I'm either in hospital or not. I flick on the radio to find out what day it is.

Hello to all you early risers on this Thursday morning!

Oh shit, it's bin day. I reverse back to put the bins out. Correction: there are no days *except* for bin day.

Two key things are causing a chatter of excitement in the staff room. One being that the overall number of Covid patients is dropping, and two, that vaccines are being given. Colleagues have been getting their first dose and mine is today. Glad to be getting it, but every now and then I twitch and rub my arm with angst as – surprising, I know – I'm really scared of needles. I spend most of my time putting them into people, much bigger than the ones used for a vaccine. Yet the idea of having a tiny, little needle in *my* arm? No. *Thank. You.* No one believes an anaesthetist can be scared of needles, but at least I'm very sensitive and aware to patients who are needle phobic. Not that it's been an issue recently, with patients not awake to tell me if they're scared of needles. Instead, I've been scared for them.

✚

I take a trip to the toilet before heading to the vaccine appointment, to lock myself away for a couple of minutes and build up the courage for an injection. As the ICU bathrooms are busy, I head off to find the nearest one, a cubicle off the main corridor, and shut myself inside. I initially don't spot the many notes stuck to the mirror in a circle, leaving a hole in the middle so they provide a halo to my tired face, with huge bin bags under my eyes. All of the pieces of paper are bright, different colours. Some have been there for a long time and are curling at the edges, others look more recent. All with messages to staff on.

We're proud of you!
You've done such a good job!
You are capable of amazing things!

I can't decide if this support is for working in Covid, having my vaccine or simply for my utilization of the facilities. I take the plaudits for all, especially the vaccine.

It doesn't feel like I'm doing something amazing or to be proud of. Doing the best I can doesn't seem like it's cutting it. Everything seems so bloody numb.

✛

'But you're an anaesthetist?' the vaccine nurse asks, surprised.

'Yes,' I say, bracing myself and looking the other way into the large hall, grimacing, while everyone else is getting their vaccine without a fuss.

'And you're scared of needles?'

'Yes.'

'Don't you spend your day putting needles in people?'

'Yes. When will it be over?'

'I put your vaccine in 30 seconds ago, you didn't even notice.'

I look back and see the nurse filling out the paperwork. I puff out my cheeks, a sigh of relief.

If working in Covid ICU has shown me anything, it's that vaccines are going to be key in returning to normal life. Prevention is most definitely better than cure, mainly because we don't have a cure. We have limited treatments that may or may not work, but it's more down to luck how people respond. No sooner is the vaccine spreading into my muscle and beyond than we receive an email that says once again anaesthetic trainees are being called back to the motherland, back to the operating theatres, back to anaesthetizing.

✚

Buoyed by the vaccine and an end to another ICU redeployment, I pull on the PPE with a little more zest than usual. The overly warm, shower curtain of a gown is comforting compared to the Baltic home set-up from earlier. I peel back the plastic sheeting to enter ICU, then look across the unit, which is completely full, as it has been for so long. But now not *just* with Covid patients, as other effects of the pandemic – patients who've attempted suicide and those with severe alcohol-caused problems – start appearing in the ward. It feels there has been such an increase in attempted suicides recently, every shift there seems to be another. The pandemic isn't just about those infected or the people that need hospitalization, it's everyone. Now and even after (if ever) coronavirus finally disappears and is consigned to the past, will there be help for people? Will there be proper support for GPs and mental-health resources so people have somewhere to turn? Will we have resources to support people recovering from this infection who suffer ongoing physical and mental-health problems?

I don't want to see patients just survive. I want them to live their lives.

✚

I can't tell you what it is I need after all this. I've been lost in a tension of just getting through days, feeling guilty for not catching up with friends or family because I'm too tired even for a call. I've just been too reliant on coffee to get me anywhere.

✚

As I start thinking about more coffee, Maria, the ICU nurse, catches me looking vacant again.

'Ah, Ed, there's a problem with the tubing system on my

ventilator, could you breathe for Sami while I change it? It'll only take five minutes.'

'Sure.'

I get up towards Sami's head among all the wires and machines. With the ICU at capacity and no spare ventilators nearby, I am the next best thing, a ventilator without the beeps. Sami is in his 40s and of slight build, with dark thinning hair. Before this, he was fit and well, but now he has been in ICU for three weeks with coronavirus and is not doing well, with all his major organs suffering. I move carefully past the dialysis machine, which takes his blood off into a machine, filters it and sends it back to him, making up for the job his kidneys can't seem to do. Moving into position, I'm careful not to dislodge any wiring or the nasogastric tube, which goes through his nose and stomach for feeding and medications.

We disconnect the ventilator from the breathing tube going into Sami's mouth. His body and breathing stops with the ventilator gone, so I attach a bag that inflates with oxygen for me to squeeze in breaths. I watch as Sami's chest rises and falls while he lies motionless. The ventilator needing Maria's attention now flashes and beeps with alarms to say:

Warning! Disconnection

Maybe I am a ventilator?

The same disconnect alarm has been going off in me since I took a phone call earlier. A relative calling.

'I just want to thank you all for looking after my dad, and just wondered where I can take some of his clothes to? He only had the hospital gown.'

'Oh. I'm so, so sorry, let me check for you.'

I wander off to find out. I have absolutely no idea.

Their father came into the unit and died in the short time I was off, and now I'm struggling to help the relatives afterwards. I've gone from talking to patients and getting to know them, to barely speaking to them, to only meeting them in a coma, or even only after they've died. It's not how I ever imagined my interactions with patients would evolve. I love talking to patients, getting to know them, building rapport and reassuring them where I can. I also love giving drugs and *not* talking to patients, but only because it's for an operation or procedure, not forever.

It's not that I *never* expect to see death. Part of the job is dealing with critically ill patients, and a lot of my future work will involve ICU. (Some people choose to specialize in both anaesthetics and ICU. Not me, thanks. There are enough exams in anaesthetics.) It's just I was used to seeing *most* patients get better, not most people die. I've gone from feeling like we can do something to feeling pretty futile, a huge change of perspective from a total belief that we can help.

✚

'Actually I need some other things, will you be OK for 15 minutes?' Maria announces, hands on hips. I raise my eyebrows and shrug to say, 'Well, I can't really disappear.'

'Thank you, doctor!' Maria wanders off.

I pan across the unit to all the patients and everyone tending to them, the usual noises, the PPE, the lack of relatives, the exhausted look on everyone's faces (or what I can see of them). The other ventilators attached to patients breathe away, all the machines looking at me, turning their mechanical noses up to an inferior human ventilator. I imagine them belittling me.

Who is this human with no range of settings and lacking any beeping noises?

I look down at Sami, using both my hands to gently squeeze in more breaths, realizing I've synchronized my own to his now. In. Out. Inspiration. Expiration.

Corpus curare spiritumque

'To care for the body and its breath of life.'

I remember seeing this motto from the Australian and New Zealand College of Anaesthetists. It feels most pertinent now as I stand here doing just that.

As Maria returns with a now-working ventilator, the bleep goes off.

Adult emergency. A&E Resus

The consultant, Hans, and I quickly strip off PPE and head towards the resuscitation room in A&E. It's a young man who suddenly collapsed in the street. The A&E runs frantic with people as some attempt to resuscitate and stabilize him while others try to find out his name. He's barely breathing for himself and isn't conscious, so Hans and I get drugs and equipment ready for an emergency intubation. The drugs go in fast, we wait a short while for them to work, looking at the clock as the seconds tick by like hours. I have a look into his mouth with my gloved fingers, the tongue flops down and I place the laryngoscope blade to move it out of the way, then glide past his teeth, into the throat until I see the pink, leaf-shaped epiglottis, the thing that stops food going into your windpipe. Sliding in a bit further, I lift up his epiglottis, exposing the opening to his windpipe. I grab the breathing tube and slide it into place between his vocal cords, then secure it and attach him to the ventilator. By the time we're ready for the scans and taking him to the unit, Worrall has come to take over from me for the night shift. I drift slowly out the door and take a look back as I leave. The patient can't be more than, what, 30?

✚

The next day is my first back in anaesthetics and there is a palpable sense of renewed, almost sustained optimism running in the theatre complex, more so than after the first wave. Conversations about operations become the main topic. Operating is stepped up, Dr Commons is walking around enthused by the place filling with familiar smells of rancid abscesses being popped or the peculiar odour of bone cement used by orthopaedic surgeons.

'MMM mmm! I *love* the smell of abscess in the morning,' he barks.

Covid-19, finally, takes a backseat.

✚

I am sent off to attend to another patient needing an abscess draining on the ward. Zahra, a middle-aged lady, sits with a book on her lap, looking up at me above her glasses. She patiently listens as I go through my spiel about why she is having a general anaesthetic for her operation. I go through the risks involved and ask if she has any questions. I realize just how much I've missed these interactions. It feels, on the back of a pandemic, that being an anaesthetist has changed fundamentally. It's not just about doing my job any more, knocking people out or being the glorified drug dispenser. There might be more coronavirus waves, or there might be another, completely unrelated pandemic. If so, anaesthetists will be one of the first to pull on the PPE and go to ICU when the going gets tough and we'll be one of the last to take it off. It's not what I want, but we'll have to do it if patients need us. It makes me value these run-of-the-mill, day-to-day moments more.

'I don't like losing control,' Zahra says at the end.

And that's exactly it. None of us have been in control. We lost it with this pandemic. Anaesthetists normally take control for their patients when they are unconscious and vulnerable. But I lost my role in Covid, lost control of being able to take care, to help people get better and recover. To an extent, we were rendered powerless.

'Losing control is exactly what happens, but I'll certainly look to give it back to you.'

She smiles and goes back to her book.

✚

Shortly after Zahra is brought down to the operating theatres, Tamsin, a trainee nurse with us today, starts hooking her up to the monitors.

I settle down next to Zahra on one knee, a sort of proposal position, and hold her hand, looking for veins to invade.

'Hmm, not a lot going on.'

'Anything I can help with?' Tamsin asks.

I spot one vein barely visible.

'Bit of support. I could do with a squeeze of the hand, please.'

The vein limply starts to bulge as I tap over it, encouraging it to pop up. Keeping my eyes on it, I reach behind me to pick up the cannula and feel something strange, tightening. I can't move. I turn to see Tamsin is now clasping my hand.

'You're doing *really* well, doctor.'

'I meant . . . squeeze Zahra's hand? To help her veins pop up?'

'Oh.' She lets go and hurriedly grabs Zahra's wrist.

I manage to thread the cannula into a vein and soon after I inject the drugs.

Zahra within seconds goes from alert and awake to unconscious. An hour later, though, she's back in control.

I, like all junior doctors, will continue to move hospitals, rotate to different places, constantly shifting my place of hospital work and life. You never stay at one hospital until you reach your end of training, but for me that is years away. It adds to the sense that medicine is just a job and a hospital is just a building. I give my best to the patients. Maybe some will remember me. The hospital you slave away at won't remember or reward you. When I leave, someone will come along and take my place. People drift away on different rotations, the friends and colleagues I've met will disperse, the ghost and team effort of coronavirus will be consigned to memories. That's why, in order to retain doctors, we need to support them, allow them a life outside of work, allow them to completely de-stress and re-energize, bringing us back fresh. To avoid burnout. Because things can get worse. They might get worse. I wince at Covid news reports from Brazil, where the horror story of running out of 'intubating drugs', aka the anaesthetic, in some hospitals is so bad they're just paralysing patients and putting breathing tubes in. This means patients are completely awake. The thought makes me nauseous at how awful it is. They are aware as someone puts a tube through their mouth, into their windpipe. They can hear and feel everything. It's unthinkable. The pandemic has led to this happening. In India, too, the health-care system is overrun, deaths are soaring, everywhere running out of oxygen. There are reminders that it could come back again, even worse.

But what more can you give?

Honestly, I don't know if there is anything I have left to give. I want to help people, want to do more for them. But I feel so helplessly numb. I feel like a cog in a machine that's fallen out onto the floor, but the machine keeps going, chugging away without me, its exhaust bellowing into my face. With so many parts bigger than tiny me, I wonder if I am wanted or even needed here? Where do I fit in? I feel overdosed on sadness.

✚

I wonder what has happened to the collapsed patient in A&E yesterday, and as I head towards ICU to find out, Sally calls me.

'Ed? Grab yourself a quick drink and come help me in theatre 3.'

I quickly drain a bottle of water, then head in to find on the operating table is the young, male patient from A&E resus yesterday, who had traumatically had an irrecoverable brain haemorrhage. His body is being kept alive for organ retrieval and the whole situation swirls around me. I don't know how any of this is done, I don't recognize any of the surgeons or retrieval team,

I don't know anything about the anaesthetic parameters or the drugs to be used. I've gone from knowing what to do to clueless in seconds.

I look at the notes to find out his name. Christopher.

'Don't worry about all this, just fill some of the charts here.' Sally hands them to me.

I start filling out anaesthetic charts, the heart rate, blood pressure, breathing volumes and more. All of them soon to be the last ever recordings. I watch as organs, one by one, are carefully removed. Heart and lungs will go, almost everything will. All to be quickly taken and given to patients in desperate need of donation. Untold sadness here will give hope to many others waiting, Christopher will save lives.

Eventually colleagues come to relieve both me and Sally, as the retrieval is set to go deep into the night, until finally the organ team have taken all they need, then all the monitoring and machines will be switched off.

Breathless.

Because, eventually, everything stops.

Chapter 16

My bleep goes off. Jeez, August 2021 and we're still using these things.

> *Emergency! Anaesthetic registrar to A&E resus!*
> *Emergency!*

Anaesthetic registrar? Wait a second, that's now me.

Shit!

Acknowledgements

A huge, humongous thank you to the amazing Romilly Morgan, my incredible and patient editor.

Thank you to my fantastic Curtis Brown agents, Alice Lutyens, Sophie and Cath, who made this all happen.

Thank you to Jo, for your constant support, assertiveness and snack provisions.

Thank you to the fantastic people at Brazen and Octopus who helped bring all this together.

To Rob Norris, for your brilliance and guidance.

To Mum and Dad (Ann and John Patrick), Johnno and the Patricks, Katy and the Emmersons, I love you all.

Thank you to Mark Goddard for being a constant rock.

Finally, thank you to Nelly for all the adventures, to Stormy for the dead animals that are apparently gifts. And Peanut, no thanks to you.

Other than my immediate family, characters, locations and incidents have been changed. Any resemblance to actual persons, living or dead is entirely coincidental.

Lyrics on page 138 from *OPM* – 'Heaven Is a Halfpipe', written by Matthew Meschery, Geoff Turney, John Edney and Roy C. Hammond

Lyrics on page 141 from *Wham!* – 'Wake Me Up Before You Go-Go', written by George Michael.

This **brazen** book was created by

Editorial Director: Romilly Morgan
Editor: Ella Parsons
Assistant Editor: Sarah Kyle
Deputy Art Director: Jaz Bahra
Cover Design: Two Associates
Photography: Chris W.R Cox Photography
Copyeditor: Sarah Hulbert
Typesetter: Jeremy Tilston
Senior Production Manager: Peter Hunt
Sales: Kevin Hawkins & Dominic Smith
Publicity & Marketing: Karen Baker & Matt Grindon
Legal: Clare Hoban, Imogen Plouviez & Sasha Duszynska Lewis